THE HOLISTIC HERB/
SUCCESSFUL STRESS

Looks at what stress is, what it does – both beneficially and problematically – and at the many ways to alleviate the effects of excess stress, with the emphasis on the use of herbs.

THE
HOLISTIC HERBAL
WAY TO
SUCCESSFUL
STRESS
CONTROL

David Hoffmann
B.Sc., M.N.I.M.H

THORSONS PUBLISHING GROUP
Wellingborough, Northamptonshire

Rochester, Vermont

First published 1986

British Library Cataloguing in Publication Data

Hoffman, David
   The holistic herbal way to successful stress
   control.
   1. Stress (Psychology)   2. Stress
(Physiology)   3. Herbs — Therapeutic use
I. Title
155.9   BF575.S75
ISBN 0-7225-1199-X

Printed and Bound in Great Britain by
Whitstable Litho Ltd., Whitstable, Kent

Contents

Are You at Ease?

STRESS – what a word to conjure with! Anxiety and tension seem to be the common experience of our people today. What a strange state we're all in. The impact of stress leaves us punch-drunk, reeling through life in a state of shock and bemusement. Is it any wonder that anxiety and tension related problems are the bulk of those that call for our doctors' attention, and our politicians' bewilderment? I wonder how the doctors themselves are doing.

If we are to look at stress, anxiety and tension in a way that shows how to come to terms with this and not be slaves to their dictates, we must give some thought to what we actually want as a positive alternative. The opposite of stress is ease, the opposite of discomfort is comfort. In these times of confusion, ease does not enter our lives by default. It must be created and invited in, a simple enough thing to do.

In this book we shall look at what stress is, what it does – both beneficially and problematically – and then how to remove the weight it lays on our shoulders. There are many ways that may help, and we shall look at some in depth. To be truly free of stress and strain, however, means being truly *free*; an enviable and rare state. However, we can all be whole within ourselves, and it is here that ease and inner freedom lie.

Transformation is in the air. It is the keynote of all we see, do and hear. Our lives are being transformed from within and without, sometimes positively growing and other times painfully changing, but everything is in flux. The purpose of our lives and the direction of society are no longer what they were, as the basis of our collective reality and beliefs changes. It is a time of chaos and crisis; a time of great stress and yet great opportunity.

In this all-embracing environment of change there is only one point of stillness and peace and that lies within our hearts. To relieve stress, anxiety and tension in any truly meaningful way involves finding one's own healing heart. To some this is God, to others our Essential Humanity. The words are unimportant but the experience is real and vital.

Herbs and Stress

One interpretation of the psychological imbalance that colours our society is that there is a deep sense of separation, of

7

alienation from our roots. Any parent will recognize the anguish in a child separated from his father or mother. What we in the 'civilized' West have done without realizing it is to alienate ourselves from our spiritual mother, Mother Earth. In other words, our unquestioned materialism has created a deep split in the collective consciousness. No wonder that our modern scourges are anxiety and fear. We have lost our roots.

Herbalism is based on relationship – relationship between plant and person, plant and planet, person and planet. Using herbs in the healing process means taking part in an ecological cycle. This offers us the opportunity to be *consciously* involved in the living, vital world of which we are part. To invite wholeness and our world back into our lives requires awareness of the remedies being used. The herbs can link us into the broader context of planetary wholeness, so that whilst they are doing their physiological/medical job, we can do ours and build on an awareness of the links and mutual relationships.

As an example, consider the treatment of a stomach ulcer with herbs or with drugs. Comfrey, Marshmallow root, Meadow-sweet and Golden-seal can all be used to soothe and heal the ulcer. The pain and discomfort go, and with the right diet and life style, the ulcers will heal and need not come back. However, there is also the chance here for the 'patient' to become aware of the way in which the environment (through plants) is actively healing him or her. Perhaps the patient can attune to the plants, visit the places where they grow, establish a deeper rapport with nature through understanding the plants' healing qualities. In this way the treatment of the ulcer becomes part of a deeper transformative process.

If drug treatment is considered in the same way, problems arise immediately. One of the frequently used drugs for problems related to over-production of stomach acid is Tagamet. This is effective by rapidly changing some of the biochemistry that leads to ulcer formation and irritation, reducing discomfort and making life more bearable. However, in the broader context it is soon evident that a moral dilemma has arisen. The chemical process used to make this drug is renowned for the pollution produced. So instead of linking in with nature's wholeness, there is an immediate relationship with nature's pain, a direct relationship between your stomach and dead fish in a polluted river. Consider also the laboratory animals that died in the development of the drug, and the dependence on a multinational pharmaceutical industry not well known for its selfless service!

Medicine can only truly ease the stress related 'diseases' if the perspectives it embraces acknowledge the social and cultural context in which the 'illness' and the desired healing takes place. It is a therapeutic and moral mistake to use herbalism to relieve a person's physical and psychological distress only for them to return to their normal lives and continue in patterns of thought, behaviour, work and culture that are the source of the dis-ease itself.

We are at home on this planet – we have only to recognize it. Through the very ills of humanity comes a clue, a signpost to this reality via the gift of herbal remedies. We are part of a wonderfully integrated whole. This is not the stuff of vague idealism and mysticism but a solid reality, the basis of this book and the whole of herbal medicine.

What is Holistic Medicine?

There is a difference between herbs, or for that matter drugs or homoeopathic remedies, and the context within which they are used. Herbalism can be practiced holistically, as can orthodox medicine and other complementary therapies, but what is holistic medicine, other than the latest 'buzz' word?

As people in all fields of life explore the implications of a holistic and ecological world view, medicine and the healing arts are to the forefront. It is now becoming possible to articulate what a holistic approach to health is, rather than the ideal of 'treating the whole person and not the symptoms'.

Holistic medicine addresses itself to the physical, mental and spiritual aspects of those who come for care, viewing health as a positive state, not as the absence of disease. It emphasizes the uniqueness of the individual and the importance of tailoring treatment to meet each person's needs. The promotion of health and the prevention of disease is a priority whilst stressing the responsibility of each individual for his or her own health. In doing this it uses therapeutic approaches that mobilize the person's innate capacity for self-healing.

Whilst not denying the occasional necessity for swift medical or surgical intervention, the emphasis is on understanding and *self-help*, on education and self-care rather than treatment and dependence. Illness may be an opportunity for discovery as well as a misfortune.

A holistic approach to health care includes understanding and treating people in the context of their culture and community. Understanding and a commitment to change those social and economic conditions that perpetuate ill health are as much a part of holistic medicine as its emphasis on individual responsibility. Most importantly, holistic medicine transforms its practitioners as well as its patients.

Such holistic perspectives suggest exciting ways in which health care can develop in Britain, but there is a need to develop the relationship between the complementary therapies and orthodox medicine. This is the way to create the framework that will fulfil expectations of health and well-being which have been raised.

To summarize, herbal medicine has much to contribute to the development of a holistic health service, using the healing plants provided by nature. The use of herbs for healing brings us immediately in touch with our world in a profoundly deep and uplifting way. Many ills of our culture stem from our sense of separation from the Earth, from the ground of our being. Herbal medicine, whilst being a valid and effective therapeutic tool, can also be part of a personal, and even social, transformation.

Stress

There can be no doubt that stress-related diseases are on the increase. Heart problems, digestive maladies, mental disturbances, all potentially stress induced, are striking people down in their thirties, forties and fifties. The tremendous increase of medical progress in recent years has not brought with it any significant overall improvement in health. It is true that great successes in the control of contagious or infectious diseases have occurred, but too much attention has been given to treatment after the fact, to intervention and cure rather than prevention.

The history of medical research has increased our understanding of disease processes, and major advances have been made in all the various branches of medicine. Now, more than ever before, the great challenge to medicine is prevention rather than cure. Beneath much of our disease today, there is a common denominator – STRESS.

The skills demanded by our jobs are changing, as are the goals and expectations of society itself. This change is happening at such an unprecedented rate that our first aim must be to learn how to cope with the stress of adaptation to change itself.

The times we live in are characterized by confusion – almost as if society is going through its adolescence! Nothing appears to have solid foundation; whether it be family relationships, the workplace, economics or international politics, there is an atmosphere of frenetic change.

Throughout this book we shall explore the many ways in which stress has an impact on our lives and how we can take back that power to live our lives in the way we want, with ease and health.

There are many different ways to define stress, and perhaps the most encompassing is: 'Stress is the response of the body to *any* demand.' It is a fundamental part of being alive and should not be avoided! The trick is to ensure that the degree of stress acting upon you is such that your life is a joy and you can *cope* with that much joy.

Just staying alive creates demands on the body for life-maintaining energy; even whilst asleep our bodies continue to function. So, from one perspective, energy usage is a basic characteristic of biological stress. Another feature of stress is its non-specificity. Any demands made upon us in daily life will bring about certain reactions in the body. The pattern of these reactions is 'stereotyped', and it will occur under a whole range of different conditions, both physical and emotional – from hot and cold to sorrow and joy. The nature of the demand is unimportant at the biological level, because the stress response is always the same.

As aware, feeling people we might see a big difference between the pain of a girlfriend leaving or the temperature dropping too fast, but to the body it's all the same!

Joy, suffering, and physical exhaustion make certain common demands upon us, which means we must adapt ourselves to something new. Various mechanisms will trigger reactions in the body under these conditions. Nervous signals are sent from the brain to several glands and these react by secreting hormones to cope with the task ahead.

So stress is not just worry and strain. As we shall see, it is a keynote of life with its ups and downs, uplifts and depressions. A new love is as much a stress as an old bank manager!

This also points out the close inter-relationship between mind and body in coping with stress-producing situations. The whole range of reactions triggered by stress starts in the brain and ends in hormonal and cellular changes, demonstrating the intricate ties that exist between the mental and physical components of who we are.

What is Stress?

It is worthwhile considering some of the scientific thought on stress. However, it may seem that much of what follows contains minor semantic differences. I'm afraid that appears to be the level of much physiological research. Bear with me for a while!

The term 'stress' can be used in a number of quite different ways. It is commonly used in three ways:

1 to describe various unpleasant situations which are considered to be stressful;
2 to describe responses which occur, in the body or mind, when an individual is confronted by an unpleasant situation (or stressor);
3 as a reflection of an incompatibility between the individual and environment.

However, in its simplest form stress is *any* pressure on the whole of us that calls for some sort of response. As has already been pointed out, the inner response is the same no matter what the stress, so let's look at what happens.

STRESS AS A STIMULUS

Stimulus-based approaches to stress are concerned with identifying aspects of the environment which have an unpleasant effect on the individual. This is a very simple view that sees human stress as the same as that studied in engineering equations, for example stresses in bridge building. The concern is with identifying stressful situations and determining how and why they have bad effects on psychology and physiology. Focus has been on work place and factors such as ambient noise levels, heat, etc. as well as job demands. Thus factors such as work under time pressure with large amounts of information to be processed are rated as stressful, as are monotony, isolation and situations where the person has little control over events.

This is fine if you think of yourself as a girder bridge, but it's not how a herbalist would view you! Some of the clear problems with this mechanistic approach to stress are:

1 Particular situations are not inherently stressful, as there are large variations in the effects of environmental stressors.
2 There are large individual differences in response to such environments. Some people thrive in the noise of a disco whilst others prefer the classical music of a string quartet.
3 There are even variations within the same individual at different times. Whether you are well rested or fatigued will determine how much of a stress roadworks are going to be on you.

It would seem that the definition of a stressful environment depends upon the response of the people involved and by what may be called 'environmental demand characteristics'. The degree of stress in a particular environment has to be seen on a spectrum. There is no doubt that walking down a motorway is very stressful, whilst sunset on the west coast of Wales has little inherent stress (unless it's June and you've got hayfever!).

STRESS AS A RESPONSE

Here stress is seen as the *response* to an adverse or 'stressful' situation. This approach is based on the work of the physiologist Hans Selye, and his general adapation syndrome (GAS), the physiology of which we shall discuss below. The theory is that the stress response is a built-in mechanism which comes into play whenever demands are placed on us and therefore is a defence reaction which has a protective and adaptive function. In other words, a general physiological reaction to all forms of stress exists, usually acting for our own good.

Simplifying, the theory suggests a three-stage process of response:
1 'Alarm' reaction.

2 'Resistance' stage which represents a functional recovery of the body to a level superior to the pre-stress state.
3 'Exhaustion', in which there is a depletion and breakdown of the rcovery of stage 2, due to continuation of stressor.

There are limitations to this inflexible physiological model of stress. It ignores the variability in response due to purely emotional or mental factors.

STRESS AS A PERCEIVED THREAT

In this interpretation, stress occurs when there are demands on an individual which she or he cannot cope with or adjust to. So stress is not associated with a specific stimulus nor a specific response, but arises when an individual perceives and evaluates a situation as threatening – when it all becomes too much.

This personal evaluation is based on an assessment of the demands of a situation and on the individual's capacity, or 'coping mechanisms', for dealing with these demands. The intensity of any threat, therefore, will depend on how well that person feels she or he can cope with the situation. Here the emphasis is placed upon how the person *perceives* the factors involved. The degree of stress is partially affected by what is going on in general, but is more intimately concerned with how that person perceives and feels. Much recent research suggests that specific situations or objects are threatening to an individual because they are *perceived* as such, rather than because of some inherent characteristic.

Bodily and Mental Responses to Stress

There is now a large body of work covering both of these aspects of response to stress. It is easier to explore them separately, but they are just different levels of analysis which need to be seen and understood in conjunction. This need to separate to ensure that the words make sense is a prime example of the way our analysis causes as many problems as it solves.

PHYSIOLOGICAL BODILY RESPONSES

The adrenal gland plays the central role in regulating physiological responses to threats or stressful demands. This is mainly, but not completely, done through the adrenal gland's central medulla, concerned as it is with immediate response, whilst the surrounding cortex is more involved in long-term responses.

The initial response – preparing the body for what has been called the 'fight or flight' reaction – involves:

1 Increased nervous-system activity, increasing heart and blood-vessel activity and allowing immediate physical exertion.
2 In conjunction, there is a release of the hormones adrenalin and/or noradrenalin into the bloodstream by the adrenal medulla. These hormones support the nervous activity through metabolic activity. The body's response to these chemicals includes:
(a) increase in heart rate and blood pressure;
(b) surface constriction of blood vessels – that means the blood will leave the skin to provide the muscles with more sugar and oxygen, which is why we go white if we're shocked;
(c) mobilization of the liver's energy stores through the release of stored glucose.

If the stress situation is very intense or continues over a period of time, the response system involving the adrenal cortex will be increasingly involved. The activity of the cortex is largely controlled by blood levels of adrenocorticotrophic hormone (ACTH) released by the anterior pituitary gland. When information about sustained stress has been 'processed' by the central nervous system a whole range of new bodily responses occur. It is these longer-term reactions that can become deleterious to the quality of life.

PSYCHOLOGICAL (EMOTIONAL/MENTAL) RESPONSES

In general terms the reaction to stress takes the following course:

1 Initially, there is an alarm and shock state which results in the hormonal and physiological changes outlined above, accompanied by emotional reactions such as anxiety or fear.
2 Individual ways of coping are activated as the person attempts to find a way of dealing with the harmful or unpleasant situation.
3 If successful the alarm reaction and anxiety state subside.
4 If the strategies fail and the stress continues to affect the person, a range of psychological reactions, including depression and withdrawal, may occur.

The implication of all this is that the consequences of failing to cope can be serious. Individuals need to develop ways of adapting to and dealing with stressful situations which suit them, and are successful for *them*.

Research into *coping* reveals that there are two broad categories of strategies. The first involves attempts to change the individual's unsatisfactory relationship with the environment, and the second contains strategies that have been described as 'palliative' as they are an attempt to soften the impact of the stress once it has occurred.

Examples of the first catagory would be:
1 Escaping from the unpleasant situation – not always possible!
2 The stress may be avoided by prior preparation for it. This could involve using skill to prepare for an exam, instead of just worrying about it. It may involve thinking through aspects of the stress situation and its likely impact, thereby preparing oneself adequately for the event. Ways of doing this will be described later.

Palliative strategies would include:
1 Denial, in which the person refuses to acknowledge all or some of the threat in the situation.
2 Intellectualization, where the individual somehow detaches herself or himself emotionally from the situation.

Both of these may serve a protective function and help the person through a difficult time with reasonable equilibrium, but there is always the danger that such strategies may make it more difficult to resolve a problem and may become established as a way of being.

For some people, other ways of coping can include escaping via the use of alcohol, tranquillizers or drugs. Even relaxation techniques can be seen in this sense of coping. All such aids to coping can have their role in some or all cases. However, the use of such coping strategies may unfortunately delay the direct action that may be needed to solve the problems.

There are some stresses for which no clear solution exists – for example, caring for the chronically ill – and in such situations softening the impact of stress may be the only way for the person to cope.

Marked emotional changes may take place following long-term or particularly severe stress. If various strategies fail, the individual may feel helpless and hopeless. He or she may regard the situation as one for which there is no solution and increasingly see himself as unable to control the events of his life. Hopelessness and helplessness are both likely to give rise to depressive feelings and may even lead to suicidal thoughts.

Following the stress of chronic illness, patients may literally give up hope and where this occurs they not only become emotionally disturbed but also appear to be more vulnerable to further physical illness.

Factors Affecting the Response to Stress

Having looked at the general physiological and psychological response patterns, it should be remembered that there is no fixed pattern of response. For any individual the pattern of response will be partially determined by many factors, some of which are listed below.

PRIOR EXPERIENCE

Specific experience of stressful situations appears to result in an improved ability to cope. The previous experience provides knowledge about a situation and puts the person into a more predictable position where he or she can be aware of how his own behaviour will affect and be affected by a potentially stressful environment – the second visit to a new doctor is always easier than the first (unless you had an argument!).

INFORMATION

Information about an impending stressful event can help preparations to ease the impact and intensity of reactions to the stress. It is well known that information describing operations and any post-operative pain can aid recovery. However, personality differences must be taken into account.

INDIVIDUAL DIFFERENCES

People differ radically in their response to the stresses associated with illness. Whilst some will cope with the demands of illness in a realistic manner, some will try and protect themselves from the full impact of the stress by *denying, playing down* or *emotionally detaching* themselves from the situation. With such people, providing information may actually increase anxiety levels.

CONTROL

Having seen that the inability to cope with stress is a basic factor, it follows that the individual's control (real or not) of a situation is an important factor. From much research it has been found that many harmful and distressing situations are those where the individual feels entirely helpless, believing that nothing he or she can do will significantly alter the outcome. This is yet another reason for power and information to be taken from the experts and put in the hands of the public.

SOCIAL SUPPORT

All that has been said so far concerns the individual. Not surprisingly, the impact of stressful events is affected by the social system the person is in. Support and empathy from others greatly softens the degrees of reaction to stress. This is especially important in early life, where many patterns of behaviour, response and perception are laid down. It seems that insufficient early social support can give rise to physical and behavioural problems, including a reduced ability to withstand stress.

Response to stress can be eased by support from the family and the community. The recovery of patients from strokes can be significantly affected by the mutual understanding or empathy shown by their families. Studies have shown that women are less likely to develop a psychiatric disorder if they have a close and confiding relationship. It is not surprising, then, that the loss of a close relationship, which represents a sudden and severe loss of support, is rated amongst the most stressful of all life events.

It says a lot about our rational and analytical approach to life that research is needed before the medical profession acknowledges that caring and support are vital parts of the healing process. Our humanity should tell us that.

Stress and Illness

From what has been said it is clear that situations that are perceived as threatening will evoke emotional responses together with coping strategies and that a whole range of bodily changes underlie the psychological changes.

It may be worth spending some time considering in greater depth the relationship between stress and illness.

PSYCHOLOGICAL FACTORS AND DISEASE

Statistical studies have shown a clear association between increased illness and the following factors:

1 Social class
2 Occupational factors

3 Life style
4 Life change or 'events'
5 Bereavement and loss.

Social class

Many of the common fatal illnesses tend to occur with higher incidence in the 'lower' social class. The reasons for this are not really understood but must include such factors as diet, smoking, housing conditions, employment/ unemployment and poorer availability of medical resources. The full ramifications of this aspect is beyond the range of this book, but security, whether financial or otherwise, is basic to any sense of well-being. A sense of personal power and the ability to have some control over one's own life are as basic to health as good diet.

Occupational factors

Some occupations, such as coal mining, carry an increased risk of physical illness. However, it is also found that some types of work, as well as the physical and social attributes of the work environment, are associated with higher levels of physical and psychological illness. A brief list of factors known to be involved includes:

1 *Shift work*, because of the disruption of circadian rhythms and social life.
2 *Long hours*, 75 hours or more.
3 *Physically adverse conditions*, cramped, noisy, bad lighting.
4 *Changes in the working environment*, to a different line of work or level of responsibility. Significantly higher levels of heart attacks occur in the year following such changes.
5 *Boring, repetitive work*, increase in frequency of depression, sleep difficulties and stomach disorders.
6 *Responsible jobs with demand and pressure*, higher risk of conditions such as high blood pressure and peptic ulceration.

Remember that these findings do not apply to all people. Many people cope quite well with adverse or demanding work environments, and may even appear to thrive. This only highlights what has been said about individual variation in response to stress. Jobs are not inherently stressful, since some people will be unaffected by them. Rather it is the difficulty in coping with the demands, changes or monotony of certain occupations which appears to make those situations unpleasant and increase the risk of ill health.

Unemployment can lead to higher risk of illness. This is brought about by the major life change and possible loss of self-esteem. What is shown here, without exploring the ramifications of unemployment, is that work meets not only financial but social and psychological needs. Failure to meet those needs will carry a high personal cost in terms of mental and physical well-being.

Life style

This will be explored more deeply later, but its clearest expression in medical terms is the type A/B personality differences. The type A personality is competitive, striving and time-pressured. This type has been called the coronary-prone behaviour pattern because of the increased chances of coronary heart disease, as opposed to the type B who would be more relaxed and calm. This is discussed in more detail in the section on heart disease.

Life change or 'events'

From a number of studies there appears to be a clear relationship between change in someone's life situation and the onset of illness. This would appear to be so because these life events require adjustments in the life pattern of an individual and this is often stressful. Such events can be anything from moving house, getting married or taking exams to being taken to court or having a car crash. These studies show that life events cluster significantly in a two-year period preceding illness and that the onset of an illness can be predicted by the number of life events. This has led to attempts to quantify the impact of life changes and the exact nature of the correlation with disease onset; these are surveyed below.

Bereavement and loss
A generalized sense of loss (actual, potential or imagined) or bereavement is a significant factor in the onset of disease. It can give rise to an emotional response of hopelessness and helplessness which results in the person literally 'giving up'. When this happens, the individual can no longer cope, psychologically and biologically, with environmental demands. If the person has a disposition to a disease, then being in this psychological state will make the disease more likely to occur because the body will be made less capable of dealing effectively with the processes which gave rise to the disease.

SOME POSSIBLE MECHANISMS
There can be no doubt that there is a definite relationship between stress and illness, but how is not understood. However, a number of ideas have been suggested. Earlier models tried to connect different illnesses with specific types of emotional conflict or personality and body types. This suggests that some sort of body builds and temperaments would be more likely to develop one physical disease under stress than others. However, there is little agreement amongst the experts.

Selye, in defining the general adaptation syndrome (GAS), has most to say on the subject. He maintains that the biological changes accompanying the GAS result in both short- and long-term adverse physical changes. These are described as *diseases of adaptation* since they are the outcome of a system of defences against threatening stimuli.

The disease process is thought to arise as the result of factors such as: (a) the physiological effect of certain hormones from the adrenal and pituitary glands; (b) the impact of the inflammation process; and (c) a general state of lowered resistance. The actual disease that manifests will depend on a range of factors including genetics, physical weakness and even specificaly learned bodily responses.

The GAS helps explain the effects of life changes or events on health. Life changes require readjustment by the individual and this could result in physiological activation. Over time this could have a deleterious effect on the body and result in illness. This would explain why more frequent and severe life changes have an increased likelihood of preceding the onset of disease. So it follows that sustained and unsuccessful attempts at coping with life will lower bodily resistance and enhance the probability of disease occurring.

How to Recognize Stress

There are many ways in which stress can show itself in a person's life, and it would be an impossible task to try and enumerate all such ways. However, when stress has reached beyond the point of being a healthy stimulant and becomes deleterious to health, it usually takes the form of what doctors call 'anxiety'. The GP may call it an anxiety attack, an anxiety neurosis or a whole range of other grand-sounding names. It means life is becoming too much of a strain. Let's look at anxiety for a moment.

Anxiety States

These include various combinations of mental and physical symptoms of anxiety occurring either in attacks (panic) or as a persisting state.

Anxiety as a concept suggests the following:
1 An emotional state coloured with the experienced quality of fear.
2 An unpleasant emotion which may be accompanied by a feeling of impending doom.
3 A feeling directed towards the future, perceiving a threat of some kind.
4 There may be no recognizable threat or one which by reasonable standards is out of proportion to the emotion it seemingly provokes.
5 There may be an experience of bodily discomfort and actual bodily disturbance.

PANIC

For some people the anxiety takes the form of occasional or recurrent attacks. These are characterized by recurrent panic attacks that occur unpredictably, though certain situations may become associated with them. It starts as a sudden onset of intense apprehension, anxiety and fear, often with a feeling of impending doom. Feelings of unreality may occur. Any of the body symptoms described below may occur. There will often be the development of 'anticipatory fear' of loss of control, so that the person becomes afraid of, for example, being left alone in public places. The anticipatory fear may itself precipitate an attack.

Symptoms of Anxiety

There is not an anxiety 'symptom' as such, but it would be worth listing the whole range of bodily signs that have been associated with tension and anxiety in general. This is given in Table 1.

Table 1: Symptoms of anxiety

Anxious mood
Worries
Anticipation of the worst
Apprehension (fearful anticipation)
Irritability

Fears
Of dark
Strangers
Being left alone
Large animals, etc.
Traffic
Crowds

Intellectual (Cognitive)
Difficulty in concentration
Poor memory

Depressed mood
Loss of interest
Lack of pleasure in hobbies
Depression
Early waking
Diurnal swing

General body sensations
Tinnitus (noises in the ear)
Blurring of vision
Hot and cold flushes
Feelings of weakness
Prickling sensations

Respiratory symptoms
Pressure or constriction in chest
Choking feelings
Sighings
Tightness of breath.

Genito-urinary symptoms
Frequency of urination
Urgency of urination
Suppressed periods
Excessive bleeding during a period
Development of frigidity

Premature ejaculation
Loss of erection
Impotence

Physiological accompaniments of behaviour
Tremor of hands
Furrowed brow
Strained face
Facial pallor
Swallowing
Belching
Sweating
Eye-lid twitching

Tension
Feelings of tension
Fatigue
Inability to relax
Startled response
Moved to tears easily
Trembling
Feelings of restlessness

Insomnia
Difficulty in falling asleep
Broken sleep
Unsatisfying sleep and fatigue on waking
Dreams
Nightmares
Night terrors

General somatic (Muscular)
Muscular aches and pains
Muscular stiffness
Muscular twitchings
Grinding teeth

Heart symptoms
Tachycardia
Palpitations
Pain in chest
Throbbing of vessels
Fainting feelings
Missing beat

Gastro-intestinal symptoms
Difficulty in swallowing
Wind
Dyspepsia: pain before/after meals,
    burning sensations, fullness,
    waterbrash, nausea, vomiting, sinking
    feeling
Burps
'Working' in abdomen
Looseness of bowels

Loss of weight
Constipation

Autonomic symptoms
Dry mouth
Flushing
Pallor
Tendency to sweat
Giddiness
Raising of hair

(From: Hamilton, M. 'The Assessment of Anxiety States by Rating' *British Journal of Medical Psychology* 32, 1959, pp 50-55)

Life Events

We needn't wait for the physical signs of stress to show themselves before we actively move towards ease in our lives. Later in the book a whole range of specific techniques will be discussed and herbal remedies suggested that will help with problems when they arise.

It is worth taking note of predictable problems before they actually arrive. To this end a study in America has produced a scale showing the impact of certain life events and this is given in Table 2. Of course, for some a particular event will be more or less of an impact than for others. Even so it provides some valuable insights.

Table 2: Life events

Life event	Value
1. Death of a spouse	100
2. Divorce	73
3. Marriage separation	65
4. Detention in jail	63
5. Death of a close family member	63
6. Major personal injury or illness	53
7. Marriage	50
8. Being fired at work	47
9. Marital reconciliation	45
10. Retirement	45
11. Major change in health or behaviour of a family member	44
12. Pregnancy	40
13. Sexual difficulties	39
14. Gaining a new family member (e.g. through birth, adoption, a relative moving in, etc.)	39
15. Major business readjustment	39
16. Major change in finances (either a lot better off or a lot worse off)	38
17. Death of a close friend	37
18. Changing to a different line of work	36
19. A major change in the number of arguments with spouse (e.g. either a lot more *or* a lot less than usual regarding children, personal habits, etc.)	35
20. Taking out a mortgage	31
21. Foreclosure on a mortgage or loan	30
22. A major change in responsibilities at work	29
23. Child leaving home	29
24. In-law troubles	29

25. Outstanding personal achievement 28
26. Wife beginning *or* stopping work outside the home 26
27. Starting or completing formal schooling 26
28. Major change in living conditions (e.g. building a new house, deterioration of home) 25
29. Change of personal habits, such as dress 24
30. Troubles with the boss 23
31. Major change in working hours or conditions 20
32. Changing to a new school 20
33. Change in the usual type and/ or amount of recreation 19
34. Major change in social activities 18
35. Taking out a loan 17
36. Major change in eating habits 15
37. Going on holiday 13
38. Christmas 12

(From: Holmes, T. and Rahne, 'The Social Readjustment Rating Scale' *Journal of Psychosomatic Research*, 11, 1967, pp. 213-18)

The relative impact of these events will be different for different people, but the overall sense is clear. In America this scale has been suggested as a tool in self-evaluation and management of stress. Dr Thomas Holmes has come up with these guidelines for its use:

1 Become familiar with the life events and the amount of change they may require.
2 With practice you can recognize when a life event happens.
3 Think about the meaning of the event for you and try to identify some of the feelings you experience.
4 Think about the different ways you might best adjust to the event.
5 Take your time in arriving at decisions.
6 If possible, anticipate life changes and plan for them well in advance.
7 Pace yourself. It can be done even if you are in a hurry.
8 Look at the accomplishment of a task as a part of daily living and avoid looking at such an achievement as a 'stopping point' or as a time for letting down.
9 *Remember*, the more changes you have, the more likely you are to get sick. The units on the scale are called 'life change units' and give some indication of the chances of getting ill in the near future:
– With more than 300 for the last year, almost 80 per cent get sick.
– With 150 to 299 about 50 per cent get sick.
– With less than 150 only about 30 per cent get sick.
So the higher the score the more you should take care of yourself!

The important point to bear in mind is that stress and the resulting tension and anxiety is sometimes predictable. Don't be a victim! Recognize that you may be moving into a particularly difficult period in your life and actively ease its impact on you.

The advice about herbs is also perfect for preventing tension building up. The herbs in question are discussed later, but also bear in mind your body's state. Should you get some exercise or a massage? Is your diet providing enough B vitamins for the extra stress? Are you in touch with whatever is meaningful for you? Should you go for more nature walks? and so on. Prepare for the pressure and thus prevent any untoward impact on you.

What to do About Stress and Anxiety

There is much that can be done to ease the impact of stress and lessen the weight of anxiety and tension that we so often carry around with us today. The key to it all is an inner attitude of taking responsibility for our own lives and the qualities with which we colour our lives. To aid the search for ease and peace in a world of confusion there are many techniques of help that we can use.

The very range of approaches and types of help that is offered today can become a stress! Where to turn, which therapy to use? Always a difficult question, especially when life is in one of its heavier times. That question may be the last that needs to be asked. In the search for inner ease, the different therapies and techniques are at best only a way of helping us to find the peace that is in us anyway.

Each of the healing techniques embodies a profound truth and a great gift of healing wisdom. However, humanity is complex indeed, and our ills are a microcosm of that complexity. There is a need to build bridges and relationships between the wisdoms and insights each therapy embodies so that a move can be made towards a more Holistic Health Service.

I shall try to do so with a simple model showing how the various approaches to health and wholeness can work together so that our deep and inner peace can become part of our waking, active life.

All holistic therapists know that healing is an expression of wholeness, health *is* wholeness and can be seen as the expression of integration that a person embodies. The emotions, thoughts and spirit are as important to health as are the organs and tissues of the body.

The person who is 'ill' is in fact also the 'healer'. Aid can be sought from 'experts', be they medical herbalists or GPs, but the responsibility for healing can never be truly handed to another. Healing comes from within and is inherent in being alive. It is our gift and our responsibility. This comes as a surprise to many, conditioned as we are these days into handing over our power to experts, but in healing, as in all life, we are free.

Healing is rarely an act of consciously harnessing inner energy, but is always a release and expression of this inner power. As a unique expression of an individual's life this healing can be facilitated by various tools and techniques. Numerous therapies have been developed throughout history that have much to offer to the healing arts. However, these do not heal. They cannot heal, they can only aid in the healing process.

The apparent multitude of healing techniques, often appearing to contradict each other, can be seen as an interrelating ecology of approaches, an ecology of therapeutics. Seeing the connections between different schools of healing makes it clear that a unique blend of therapies may ideally suit one person whilst a different blend would be right for someone else. The key to health and wholeness in each case is finding what will evoke the innate inner ease that is our gift as living people. This may be with medical techniques or a change in social and spiritual factors. The model does not deny the fundamental importance of understanding pathological disease processes. Rather it recognizes that to be human is much more than simple biological functioning. This provides us with a choice as to the best way to aid the movement to stillness within.

Four branches of healing techniques can be identified: *medicine, body work, psychotherapies* and methods of *spiritual integration*. Each of these branches consists of several specific therapies. But whilst having profound specific actions, these will only heal and help if in that unique individual it will work to promote the inner process of being at ease. I have tried to show this in Figure 1.

The relationships shown in the diagram are limited by being shown as two-dimensional. Each of the therapeutic approaches mentioned can be related to each other. The model is one of a geodesic web of related therapies

that may be called into play to facilitate the central core of self-healing and peace. Many of the therapies can be placed in more than one of the four branches shown, and while the whole model has major limitations, a pattern of relationship is highlighted and this is the vital point.

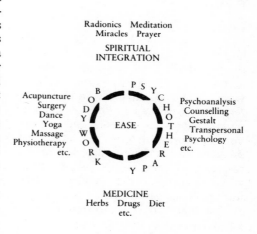

Figure 1 The four branches of healing techniques

Medicine

Medicine may be identified as anything that is taken, and may include herbs, chemical drugs, homoeopathic remedies, diet, Bach flower remedies, aromatherapy, etc. It may seem strange to group drugs and herbs together, but as 'things' they are all part of the diversity and richness of our planet. Whether it be hydrocortisone, Meadow-sweet or a Bach flower remedy, all are produced from the body of the earth in one way or another, and by taking them we cycle them in that planetary body. There is nothing universally bad about drugs or universally good about herbs. Let us be thankful for the choice. The use of drugs to stop a biochemical disease process is at times valid and life-saving, but in the context of this model that is only partial healing. Holistic practitioners know that the removal of symptoms is not the same as being healed.

Body Work

Body work recognizes that the physical body has a deep wisdom far outstretching the mind's ability to comprehend. A vast range of techniques are available, with surgery as perhaps the most mechanical and invasive. This does not deny its undoubted power in saving and enhancing life, but points out the limitations inherent in a technique that is purely a response to already established pathology. However, we have many other, less rigorous body-work approaches. Acupuncture offers a profound way of balancing body energies and, as the Chinese experience shows, it has a lot to offer in combination with herbal treatment. To these major therapies, very different approaches to the body must be added: manipulative methods, such as osteopathy, chiropractic and physiotherapy. I do not want to debate the pros and cons of each therapy here but to begin the painting of a broad picture of relationships between them, and physiotherapy must be included here. In the context of stress management some of the body-work tools take on a primary role. These include yoga, Alexander Technique, Feldenkrais, exercise and dance. Massage, with its many variations, has a wonderful contribution to make but the list of names would be almost endless here!

Psychotherapy

Psychotherapy and counselling are increasingly relevant in our stressed and insane times. Much pain and trauma is the result of emotional and mental problems which are approachable through the techniques developed to enhance inner knowing and psychological integration. These may be the traditional, but limited, approaches of psychoanalysis or the more holistically orientated techniques of humanistic and transpersonal psychology such as gestalt and psychosynthesis. The experience of the growth movement with its great proliferation of techniques has much to offer in a broad approach to healing. The work of counsellors in our society is greatly undervalued.

Spiritual Integration

For the spiritually orientated it can be said that dis-ease is the result of an inhibited soul life. Without exploring the implications of that, all holistic medical practitioners would recognize the importance of techniques of spiritual integration. Inherent in a holistic view of humanity is the perception of an integrating centre, a spiritual core, a source of life and love. In approaching human spirituality from the angle of healing, there are ways in which we can open to our higher selves, and ways in which others can affect our 'spiritual bodies'. Examples of possible ways to do this would be through prayer or some variety of meditation, spiritual healing, radionics, etc. It is here that I would include the mystery of 'miracles', the undoubted miraculous healing of incurable conditions. The implications of this go way beyond the focus of this book, but let us thank God that they are real! This mutually supportive network of therapies and techniques provides a spectrum of insights that recognize that individuals are unique. Each person may find a different approach, or group of approaches, more beneficial than others. For some it may be the trio of herbal medicine, osteopathy and psychotherapy that gives the most help in their attempts to be healthy and whole, whilst for others it may be surgery and drugs. All are valid in the search for the key that releases self-healing and inner peace.

This attempt to understand the relationships and to build bridges is but one example of a whole transformation taking place within Western intellectual life. We live in times of chaos and transformation out of which a whole new paradigm, or pattern, of world view is slowly emerging. This small model attempts to show the relationship between therapies and is but a part of a greater vision that is holistic healing.

These are some of the many ways to help in the movement to inner ease and to manage stress, anxiety and tension. We shall consider what each has to offer and then look at ways of using them in practice.

The main approach we shall consider is *herbalism*, but will also cover *relaxation therapy, meditation, yoga, autogenic training, biofeedback, diet, dance, massage* and many others. They will be considered in the context of the four branches of healing arts described above.

Medicines

We shall start our review of the ways to manage stress and relieve anxiety and tension by examining things that can be *taken*. *Herbal* medication will be looked at in depth. Other therapies described here will be *Bach flower remedies, aromatherapy, homoeopathy* and *nutrition*.

All that is said in this section complements that given in the sections on body work, psychological techniques and spiritual integration. Stress must be approached on a broad front so that ease is a whole experience.

Herbs

Herbs have been used as medicines for as long as humanity has been aware of anything and made written records. Every culture at every point in time has based its healing arts on plants. It is only very recently that Western approaches to medicine have moved to a one-sided scientific view of illness which has seen the development of chemical medicine. In this context herbal remedies are seen as sources of valuable 'active ingredients'. This turns the dandelion into a bag of chemicals, the violet into 'raw' material.

Plant remedies are nature's gift to a suffering humanity – an expression of our belonging to the world. In these days of isolation from each other and nature it comes as an almost revolutionary thought that humanity's oneness with nature can take particular form. We have become so accustomed to 'health' coming from a bottle of pills, that the idea of a wayside plant helping in times of trauma sounds too simple to be true.

There are many ways of looking at herbs and the question of why they should work. For many people it is enough that they do! Intuition and the ineffable sense of wonder that nature draws out of us opens all but the most rationally limited mind to this possibility: that herbs can help! It is possible, however, to use the wonderful insights of science to suggest a pattern of the relationships involved. To do this we must dip into the realms of geology, evolutionary biology and spiritual ecology.

The Gaia Hypothesis and Herbal Remedies

New insights into the workings of our planet *as a whole* point to exciting perspectives within which to see ourselves. The work of the geochemist Jim Lovelock has shown us that the earth is not a passive geophysical object but an active participant in the creation of its own story – a living being that he named GAIA after the Greek earth goddess. Lovelock has described Gaia as:

> . . . a complex entity involving the earth's biosphere, atmosphere, oceans and soil; sthe totality constituting a feedback system which seeks an optimal chemical and physical environment on this planet. The maintenance of relatively constant conditions occurs through *active control* . . .

What this all implies is that our world is working actively as a whole to create and maintain optimum conditions for life to thrive and evolve. There is a recognition that human consciousness is an integral part of the evolutionary drive, and that the opportunity lies before us to embrace fully our role within the greater being of Gaia, our world. This realization is not new; it is the gift to humanity from the mystics of all ages, but the point has now been reached where these insights are the stuff of science, where the 'spiritualization of the mundane' is happening.

Ecology is showing us how all that lives upon our planet is integrated and mutually dependent in a profound and complex way. With the concept of Gaia in mind, evolution becomes an exercise in co-operation as much as competition, both processes creating the complex tapestry of today's ecology. The eco-system can only be understood as a whole. It is a self-maintaining unit, with all that is needed by any part of the whole being supplied by it. In fact, it has to be supplied by the system as there is nothing outside it. For example, we get neither Meadow-sweet nor Penicillin from outside of the earth. If the system does not take care of itself, it is not viable and so will not survive. Humanity has survived and flourished without drug therapy and the wonders of high technology surgery, and yet still produced empires, great art and the very science that has given us modern medicine.

Active Ingredients or Whole Plants?

Healing has largely been based on herbal medicine and science is now showing the chemical basis of this. One of the many ways in which Gaia circulates energy and life throughout the planet is through food and the biochemicals in food. Herbal medicines contain what are called *secondary plant products:* complex chemicals that play no apparent role in the life of the plant. Until recently, biochemists concluded that these were elaborate waste-disposal systems, but this seems totally out of keeping with the genius of plants for efficiency and design. These chemicals are the very ones that have such a marked action on human physiology.

This is not merely a fortuitous accident, but the hallmark of Gaia, evidence of a planetary circulation of energy, life and healing. By eating plants or drinking herb teas we link into a circulatory system within the biosphere and to the energy source of the sun. The secondary plant products are taking part in this planetary circulation, helping humanity and thus the health of the whole planet. Through plants, as food or medicine, we link in with the vitality of our world.

These valuable and potent chemicals are what pharmacists consider as the active ingredients of the plants. Vast funds go into the search for new potential drugs. This is not how the medical herbalist sees them nor is it the best way to harness nature's gifts. Perhaps some examples will clarify this.

Isolation and synthesis of isolated active ingredients, such as aspirin from Willow Bark and digoxin from Foxglove, is a mistake and may even be harmful. In plants these powerful constituents are balanced and made accessible to the body by the numerous other constituents present. The Chinese herb Ma Huang ((*Ephedra sinica*) contains an alkaloid called ephedrine which, in addition to its use in conditions such as asthma, raises blood pressure if given as an extracted drug. In the whole plant, however, there are six other alkaloids, the main one of which actually prevents a rise in blood pressure and an increase in heart rate. The isolated drug is dangerous, but the whole plant is balanced by nature to make a safer remedy. This raises the question of why the chemists don't extract all seven alkaloids? They clearly don't trust nature's own skills in balancing herbal remedies! Dandelion leaves are a potent and useful diuretic but require none of the usually essential potassium supplements given with conventional drug diuretics, which have potassium loss as their side-effect. The leaves are so rich in this essential mineral that dandelion leaves are a perfectly balanced remedy, leaving the body with a healthy net increase in potassium.

This reveals the core of the benefit of herbal remedies when treating stress and anxiety. Not only do remedies contain 'active ingredients' to calm the nerves or lift depression; therse things are done by gently aiding the *whole* body to be at ease and regain health.

Can a person be reduced to the level of molecules and can anxieties be interpreted as purely biochemical phenomena? Of course not. The use of potent drugs will suppress and block the expression of tension but not do anything about causes. Humanity surpasses description in the beauty and dynamic complexity of form and function, in potential and creativity. On the level of physical form the body is indeed biochemical, but its organization transcends the realms of chemical medicine. Even if the molecular complexities were comprehended, we would not be any nearer to knowing what makes us human. There is a powerful, integrating force at work within us – call it life, vital force or the spark of life. It is us and is involved with the whole of us on all levels, not just biochemical!

Herbal medicine recognizes the life force at work within us and uses the planet's gift of herbs to augment this force, bringing about a deep healing and not simply the relief of symptoms.

The Nervous System

In no other system of the body is the connection between the physical and the psychological aspects of our being as apparent as in the nervous system. Clearly, the tissue of the nervous system is part of the physical make-up of the body and, just as clearly, all psychological processes take place in the nervous system. Therefore, if there is dis-ease on the psychological level, it will be reflected in the physiological. One wonders why the physical side of being was ever regarded as separate from the psychological.

A holistic approach to herbal healing acknowledges this interconnectedness, and regards nervous tissue and its functions as a vital element in the treatment of the whole being.

Orthodox medicine tends to reduce

psychological problems to the mere biochemical level, and assumes that 'appropriate' drugs will sort out or at least hide the problem sufficiently to allow 'normal' life to continue.

Interestingly enough, some techniques in the field of complementary medicine assume or imply the other extreme, namely that psychological factors are the cause of *any* disease and that treatment of the psyche is the *only* appropriate way of healing, and will take care of any physical problem.

By bringing these two reductionist views together, we come closer to a holistic approach. With herbal medicine we can treat the nervous system as part of the whole body. We can feed and strengthen it, helping the psyche. For our being to be truly healthy, we have to take care of our physical health through the right diet and life style, but we are also responsible for a healthy emotional, mental and spiritual life. The emotional atmosphere we live in should be fulfilling, nurturing and support emotional stability. Our thoughts should be creative and life-enhancing, open to the free flow of intuition and imagination; not conceptually rigid. And, equally, we have to stay open to the free flow of the higher energies of our soul, without which health is impossible.

Any dis-ease that manifests in the body must be seen in an emotional, mental and spiritual, as well as a physical, context. We must also remember that as part of the greater whole of humanity we are, in a deep and mysterious way, connected with humanity's diseases, and immersed in a sea of impulses and factors not directly under our control. Many neuroses met in today's Western society are quite possibly normal responses to an absurdly abnormal environment, *sane* reactions of the psyche and emotions to the *insanities* of a diseased society.

In this sense, there is a limit to the healing of an individual, when the disease is really a reflection of society's disease. To be a healer in the late twentieth century involves an awareness of the whole and a certain amount of political insight, if not activity.

For us to be whole, our society must be whole. For our society to be whole *we* must be whole. For our society to truly reflect our highest aspirations, *we* have to live, embody and reflect those aspirations.

Herbal medicine can be an ecological and spiritually integrated tool to aid the nervous system of humanity, so that humanity can help itself. It is an ideal counterpart on the physical level for therapeutic techniques on the psychological level, to help people to embrace their wholeness.

Herbs for the Nervous System

There are a number of ways in which herbs can benefit the nervous system in addition to the rather simplistic ones of stimulation and relaxation. Herbal remedies that are mentioned here in a broad context are discussed in depth in the herbal section of the book.

In Western herbalism today it is common to differentiate between three kinds of herbs that act on the nervous system, or *nervines*. These are *nervine tonics, nervine relaxants* and *nervine stimulants*. It may be superfluous to point this out again, but any successful treatment of anxiety and tension problems with herbs will involve treating the whole body and not simply the signs of agitation and worry. Of course the agitation can be reduced greatly, but the whole system must be strengthened in the face of the storm!

NERVINE TONICS

Perhaps the most important contribution herbal medicine can make in the whole area of stress and anxiety is in strengthening and 'feeding' the nervous system. In cases of shock, stress or nervous debility, the nervine tonics strengthen and restore the tissues directly; there is no need to resort to tranquillizers or other drugs to ease anxiety or depression. In many 'nerve' problems, the nervine tonics can be invaluable.

Surprising as it may seem, one of the best and certainly the most widely applicable remedy to feed nervous tissue is the common Oat, which can either be taken in the form of tinctures, combined as needed with relaxants, stimulants or any other indicated remedy, or can simply be eaten as porridge. The Oats must be old-fashioned whole oat groats cooked as porridge. Instant or rolled oatflakes do not have their original integrity, and become useless here.

In a similar way to Oats, there are two remedies that have a profound action upon the body as a whole. These are Ginseng and Siberian Ginseng.

The term 'adaptogen' has been coined to describe their undoubted ability to aid the whole of the body and mind to cope with demands made upon it.

Other nervine tonics that have, in addition, a relaxing effect include Damiana, Scullcap, Vervain and Wood Betony. Of these Scullcap is often the most effective, particularly for problems related to stress.

NERVINE RELAXANTS

In cases of stress and tension, the nervine relaxants can help a lot to alleviate the condition. They are the closest natural alternative for the straight nerve tranquillizers, but should always be used in a broad holistic way. Too much tranquillizing, even that achieved through herbal medication, can in time deplete and weigh heavily on the whole nervous system.

The following list is far from complete but includes the main restoratives of the nervine relaxant category:

Black Cohosh	Lemon Balm
Black Haw	Lime Blossom
Californian Poppy	Mistletoe
Chamomile	Motherwort
Cramp-bark	Pasque-flower
Hops	Passion-flower
Hyssop	Rosemary
Jamaican Dogwood	St John's Wort
Lady's Slipper	Scullcap
Lavender	Valerian

As can be seen from this list, many of the relaxants also have other properties and can be selected to aid in related problems. This is one of the great benefits of using herbal remedies to help in stress and anxiety problems. The physical symptoms that can so often accompany the ill-ease of anxiety may well be treated with herbs that work on the anxiety itself.

In addition to the herbs that work directly on the nervous system, the *anti-spasmodic* herbs – which affect the peripheral nerves and the muscle tissue – can have an indirect relaxing effect on the whole system. When the physical body is at ease, ease in the psyche is promoted. There are anti-spasmodic herbs that relax and ease different tissues of the body. It is worth studying this book's herbal to see which herbs have this action in addition to their main one. Many of the nervine relaxants have this anti-spasmodic action, but by far the most important and safe that we should note are Cramp-bark, Valerian and Wild Haw.

The demulcents can also help in conjunction with nervines, as they soothe irritated tissue and promote healing.

NERVINE STIMULANTS

Direct stimulation of the nervous tissue is not very often needed in our times of hyperactivity. In most cases it is more appropriate to stimulate the body's innate vitality with the help of nervine or even digestive tonics, which work by augmenting bodily harmony and thus have a much deeper and longer-lasting effect than nervine stimulants.

In the last century much more emphasis was placed by herbalists upon stimulant herbs. It is, perhaps, a sign of the times that our world is supplying us with more than enough stimulus.

When direct nervine stimulation *is* indicated, the best herb to use is the Kola Nut, although Coffee, Mate Tea and Black Tea should also be remembered. A problem with these commonly used stimulants is that they have a number of side-effects and can themselves be involved in causing many minor psychological problems such as anxiety and tension. Like the other nerve stimulants mentioned above, short-term use is appropriate at times. Daily cups of strong coffee cause too many problems to list!

Some of the herbs rich in volatile oils are also valuable stimulants, one of the commonest and best being Peppermint.

The bitter herbs can have a positive effect on the nervous system through their general stimulation of metabolism and physiology. Such herbs as wormwood and mugwort come to mind.

HERBAL ALLIES

From this apparently huge and confusing list of effective remedies the appropriate ones need to be selected. Each person is going to find out that there is a particular herb that suits them very well indeed. The degree of matching may even go beyond the stated indications for the plant in any herbal that may be consulted. Such herbs have been called 'herbal allies'. There is no way of giving instructions about how to find your 'ally'. Sometimes we find them and sometimes not. If found, they act in a deep and profound way that is especially helpful in easing the impact of stress and general anxiety, let alone any specific health problems the person may have.

Daily Use of Herbal Remedies for Stress

If it is known that a period of stress and strain is about to descend and fill your life with its usual basket of goodies, it is worth recognizing this beforehand. There are certain herbs, diet and life-style changes that will minimize the impact.

In a previous chapter we discussed life events. By anticipating them it is possible to prepare in many ways, but here we shall discuss herbal aids.

There are a number of herbs that will help as gentle relaxants for regular use. They can be used as teas, as cold drinks, as relaxing foot baths, infused in massage oil, or even as full baths. The remedies can make quite delicious wines, but it could be a very herbal way to become alcoholic so they should be used with discretion. The different ways of using the herbs are described in detail in the chapter on preparations and pharmacy.

It may be best to list the plants that can be used as safe daily easers of stress and calmers of anxiety. Choose the ones for yourself by their effect on *you*. Taste and general intuition may tell which would be the most suitable to use. All those suggested are safe and are not tranquillizers. This is a partial list. The herbal section at the end of the book contains much more detailed information.

Balm
A very traditional English herb that graced Elizabethan gardens and would suit city window-boxes. Not only is it visually aesthetic but has an aroma that is strongly reminiscent of Lemon and Geranium. This is imparted into the tea and is partially responsible for the action of the herb. In addition to its relaxing action it settles the stomach and most mild digestive upsets.

Chamomile
A popular relaxing herb that has many beneficial properties on the digestion as well. It is an acquired taste.

Lavender
A wonderful herb in all ways. The very fact that nature has evolved this plant should give us the hint that underneath all our problems life is very good indeed!

Lime Blossom
A valuable and pleasant tea for easing and relaxing the stresses of the day. It acts on the circulatory system and is good for people with high blood pressure.

Oats
It may seem surprising that this food should be in a list of herbs, but remember that our food could be our medicine. Oats should be an inherent part of the diet for people under stress. They can be considered as nerve food.

Scullcap
A much stronger relaxing remedy that can be used if greater relaxation is needed.

Valerian
Stronger again and discussed in more detail later.

Wood Betony
One of our common wild herbs that will ease away daily tensions and especially those that cause headaches.

In addition to herbal remedies it is important that your food is feeding you well and this especially applies to the nervous system. In addition to all the guidelines for good diet given later, this is a time when a vitamin supplement may be required. A daily supplement of the B complex of vitamins, perhaps one combined with vitamin C, would be most beneficial. Without wanting to advertise I can strongly recommend a tablet called *Stress-B-Vite* made by American Nutrition. If this is not available then any of the other excellent preparations available today would be suitable.

Apart from healthy responses to stress – enjoying herbs and improving diet – try and see if the stress itself can be reduced. This is occasionally impossible but surprisingly often quite possible. Don't just put up with something or someone because they are there. You can change and you can change your life. It helps to re-evaluate your choices. Are you doing what you really want to do? If not, what is it that you would like to do? Give yourself permission to ask some searching questions of yourself and about your life style. Don't censor any of the answers that may come up!

After checking our your inner motivation you have the choice of what you do with it. If changing the apparent cause is too difficult or painful – well, you are free to not change it as well. With herbs and, perhaps, counselling it will be possible to ease the strain and live a less tense and anxious life. However, if you choose to change, then herbal medicine if used wisely will aid you in the process of transformation.

So from all of this it is clear that the daily use of herbs to help with the stresses and strains of daily life have much to offer. Give them a try.

When Stress Continues for a Long Time

The borderline is blurred between this degree of stress impact and the daily levels we all seem to put up with. For a gentle soul with a not too strong constitution it will be sooner than for the stronger one who copes well. Neither of these extremes of personality is 'better' than the other, we just live in a world of human diversity. That's sometimes a joy and sometimes the cause of the strain itself!

The advice given above still holds here, but in addition there are two remedies that should become staples. Not both together, but the one that is most suitable for the person concerned.

The remedies in question are Ginseng and Siberian Ginseng. As it happens, there is no close botanical relationship; the similarity in names comes from commercial interests. Of these two, perhaps Siberian Ginseng is of widest relevance, aiding and supporting the whole of the hormonal system that deals with the impact of stress.

Immediate Relief

There are times in most people's lives when things get too much and the pain of existence builds to a crescendo. At such times herbs can only be an aid, a part of a whole approach to the difficulties being faced. These difficulties can be so multifarious in our crazy and chaotic times that I shall simply talk about herbs that can be used. It may be appropriate to seek aid from the various caring professions, go on holiday or retreat, or even go to hospital.

Immediate herbal relief may be needed in a whole range of traumatic situations – from being involved in a car accident to some personal emotional crisis. In all cases the herbs will take the edge off the intensity but will rarely remove it. Pain, physical and emotional, appears to be part of the gift of our being human.

There are plants that will ease such intensity but in our society they are considered dangerous and are restricted drugs, and as such will be ignored here.

The guidelines given for the use of herbs in alleviating anxiety and tension all stand here, but the following remedies should be considered:

Jamaican Dogwood
A pain reliever, reduces anxiety and will help relaxation and sleep.

Lady's-slipper
This remedy is also called American Valerian as it has similar properties.

Passion-flower
A good and safe remedy that will help with sleeplessness. It doesn't increase passion!

Valerian
A widely applicable and quite strong relaxing plant. With some sensitive people

it has been known to cause the reverse, agitation. If it suits you, use it as strongly as you like. It is also a sleep inducer at high dosage. It will ease pain and help with digestive wind.

Wild Lettuce
This is not the common lettuce! The strength of this remedy varies from plant to plant, unfortunately. Will act as a mild tranquillizer.

Anti-spasmodic drops
These are a combination of herbs, not all nervines, that ease shock and trauma. There are a number of proprietary makes available and it is easier to buy a bottle from a reputable herb supplier than try and concoct them yourself. One of the best is that made by Potter's Ltd. Leyland Mill Lane, Wigan, Lancashire, WN1 2SB. The remedy can safely be used to ease the trauma of a shock. Take as directed on the label.

Rescue Remedy
This is discussed in more detail in the section on Bach flower remedies, but it is one of the best treatments for shock available.

Let us now move on to consider other types of medicines, that is 'things' that can be taken, apart from traditional herbal remedies.

Aromatherapy
The fragrance of flowers is one of their most wonderful gifts to humanity, and in recent years the healing value of this aroma has been increasingly acknowledged.

As with the very best of herbal medicine, the oils are beautiful things. Nature provides us with a healing that is aesthetic and uplifting even before we start using it! Whether it is looking at a flower, walking through a meadow or smelling an aromatic oil, the subtler aspects of Gaia, of Nature, are at work healing and showing us how whole we really are.

The plant's oils are the basis of the aroma and are called essential oils. Chemically each plant has an amazing array of different specific oils that combine to produce the unique quality of each type of flower. Research has shown that they have a distinct effect upon the mind as well as their antiseptic and other properties.

Aromatherapy, the use of essential oils, is a vast field and anyone interested in studying further will find recommended books in the bibliography. Here, we shall just briefly consider the oils that may help in easing anxiety and tension and the ways in which they may be used.

This therapy could be considered under the body section as the oils are usually applied to the skin in massage. However, they work through absorption by the skin and their internal effect so we shall look at them as 'medicines'.

The oils may be used for the whole spectrum of ills that a human falls prone to, from physical to mental and stress problems. Many oils have strong antiseptic and anti-bacterial properties. The application of Chamomile and Lavender oils to infected wounds can be as effective as the use of phenol. Eucalyptus sprayed in the air will purify it and has a role in any sick-room. As examples of essential oils for psychological problems we can consider Orange Flower for anxiety, worry or insomnia; Rose for stress and depression (it also has a reputation for hangovers!); Basil, Rosemary and Patchouli can stimulate mental clarity, concentration and memory.

Essential oils will be most effective if used as part of a whole programme of regaining ease. The oils should *never* be used internally unless under the guidance of a skilled medical herbalist or aromatherapist.

Each of the oils mentioned below has a vast range of actions; however, here we shall just mention their use in stress and anxiety related problems. It is a brief selection only, as nature is truly abundant in her gifts.

Basil
A refreshing and stimulating oil, it is a nerve tonic that aids concentration and clarifies the mind.

Chamomile
Soothing and calming for anxiety. For insomnia use in a late bath. Will relax muscles as well being anti-inflammatory.

Clary Sage
A good relaxing oil with euphoric effects on sensitive people! May help with insomnia.

Hyssop
A mild sedative and general nerve tonic. Helps regulate blood pressure, whether high or low.

Jasmine
A wonderful aroma that is anti-depressant and supposedly a sensual stimulant. It eases pain in the whole of the female reproductive system.

Lavender
If you only get one oil, let it be lavender! It relaxes and eases aches and pains. It has a whole range of positive physical actions but is especially useful for migraines and headaches.

Marjoram
Useful for anxiety, grief and insomnia as well as easing muscular, menstrual and rheumatic pains. May help in migraine. A very warming remedy.

Orange Flower Absolute
A beautiful strong aroma that is quite effective for anxiety and its associated symptoms such as palpitations. It will ease depression as well. Good for shock and fear.

Patchouli
A stimulant to the nerves that lifts anxiety and depression. Has a reputation as an aphrodisiac.

Pine
Primarily an antiseptic oil, but helps clear the mind and of benefit in mental fatigue.

Rose
Very soothing for the nerves and an anti-depressant. It can calm anger and alleviate hangovers.

Rosemary
An invigorating oil which may stimulate a weak memory and general dullness. Helpful for headaches.

Sandalwood
A stilling and refreshing oil that eases anxiety and nervous tension.

Verbena
An excellent nerve tonic that eases and strengthens at the same time. For all anxiety problems, especially palpitations and dizziness. An insect repellent.

Ylang-Ylang
A sweet exotic scent that is supposedly aphrodisiac. It stimulates the senses and brings about a sense of well-being. It is good for anxiety, tension and anger.

HOW TO USE ESSENTIAL OILS
As already pointed out, while they

should not be used internally, there is a whole range of ways to get the benefit of these wonderful oils.

Massage oils
These aromatic oils blend well with any bland massage oil. This gives the opportunity to experiment and learn what is most appropriate for you. An example would be 10–12 drops of essential oil to 20 ml of almond oil, or 60 drops to 100 ml of almond oil.

Bath oils
Add 5–10 drops of oil to a full bath. This way you absorb through the skin but also by inhaling.

Perfumes
Any of the pleasant fragrances may be used as perfumes, alone or blended.

Vaporization
A few drops on a heat source, such as a radiator or small bowl of hot water. All the oils evaporate easily.

Toilet water
Take 3 drops of essential oil and add to 100 ml of distilled water. Keep the mixture in a dark airtight bottle. This will keep fresh for a few weeks.

These are the best methods to help with stress problems. There are more ways of using the oils for getting rid of infections and easing muscular pains.

Bach Flower Therapy
The Bach flower remedies represent an approach to herbalism that is an alchemical amalgam of the spiritual essence of the flower in co-operation with the emotional/mental need of the person. So just as in aromatherapy it could have been included in body therapies, the Bach remedies have a place in the spiritual treatments.

They are not used directly for physical illness, but for the individual's worry, apprehension, hopelessness, fear, irritability, etc. As we have seen, the state of someone's psychic state has a major bearing on the causation, development and cure of any physical illness. The remedies appear to work with the life-force, allowing it to flow freely through or around the block and so speed healing and a return to wholeness.

Thirty-eight remedies were developed by the late Dr Edward Bach (1880–1936). The story of how he found them is wonderful indeed and worth reading about. The contact address for any information about the remedies is: Dr E. Bach Centre, Mount Vernon, Sotwell, Wallingford, Oxon, OX10 OPZ. In USA it is: Ellon (Bach USA), 463 Rockaway Ave, Valley Stream, NY 11580.

He found 38 flowers to cover the negative states of mind from which we so often suffer, categorizing them under seven major headings with further subdivisions. These headings are *apprehension, indecision, loneliness, insufficient interest in circumstances, oversensitivity, despondency and despair, over-care for others.*

These flower remedies are ideal for self-use and again much more information and supplies are obtainable from the Centre. They are inherently benign in action, have no unpleasant reactions and can be used by anyone. The dose is simply a few drops of the special extracts in water.

I shall quote from a brief guide produced by the Centre to give an idea of the uses of the remedies:

Agrimony: For those who suffer inner torture which they try to hide behind a façade of cheerfulness.
Aspen: For apprehension and forebod-

ing. Fears of unknown origin.

Beech: For those who are arrogant, critical and intolerant of others.

Centaury: Weakness of will in those who let themselves be imposed upon and become subservient, who have difficulty in saying 'no'.

Cerato: Those who doubt their own judgement and overly seek the advice of others. Often influenced and misguided.

Cherry Plum: For a fear of mental collapse, desperation or loss of control. Vicious rages.

Chestnut Bud: A refusal to learn by experience and continually repeating the same mistakes.

Chicory: Over-possessive and demanding attention. Selfishness. For those who like others to conform to their standards. Will often make martyrs of themselves.

Clematis: Indifferent, inattentive, dreamy and absent-minded. Mental escape from reality.

Crab Apple: A cleanser for those who feel unclean or ashamed of ailments. For self-disgust and the house-proud.

Elm: Temporarily overcome by responsibility or inadequacy, although normally very capable.

Gentian: Despondent, easily discouraged and dejected.

Gorse: Extreme hopelessness.

Heather: For people who are obsessed with their own troubles and experiences. Poor listeners.

Holly: For those who are jealous, envious, revengeful and suspicious. For those who hate.

Honeysuckle: For those with nostalgia who constantly dwell in the past. Also homesickness.

Hornbeam: Procrastination, 'Monday morning' feeling.

Impatiens: Impatience and irritability.

Larch: Despondency due to lack of self-confidence. An expectation of failure so they fail to make an attempt. They feel inferior although they have the ability.

Mimulus: Fear of known things, shyness and timidity.

Mustard: Deep gloom that descends for no known reason but which can lift just as suddenly. Melancholy.

Oak: Determination. Struggles on in illness and against adversity despite setbacks. A plodder.

Olive: Exhaustion – drained of energy – everything is an effort.

Pine: Feelings of guilt. They blame themselves for mistakes of others and feel unworthy.

Red Chestnut: Excessive fear and over-caring for others held dear.

Rock Rose: Terror, extreme fear or panic.

Rock Water: For those who are hard on themselves, rigid-minded and self-denying.

Scleranthus: Uncertainty, indecision and vacillation.

Star of Bethlehem: For all the effects of bad news or fright following an accident.

Sweet Chestnut: Anguish of those who have reached the limits of endurance and absolute dejection.

Vervain: Over-enthusiasm, over-effort and straining. Fanatical.

Vine: Dominating, inflexible, ambitious and autocratic. Arrogance.

Walnut: A protection remedy from powerful influences and helps adjustment to any transition or change, e.g. menopause or divorce.

Water Violet: Proud, reserved, 'superior'.

White Chestnut: Persistent unwanted thoughts. Preoccupation with a worry or event. Mental arguments.

Wild Oat: Helps determine one's intended path in life.

Wild Rose: Resignation, apathy. For drifters who accept their lot, making little effort for improvement.

Willow: Resentment and bitterness, with a 'poor me' attitude.

RESCUE REMEDY: A combination of *Cherry Plum, Clematis, Impatiens, Rock Rose, Star of Bethlehem.* An all-purpose emergency composite for causes of trauma, anguish, bereavement, and any stress.

Rescue Remedy is to treat the effect that a sufferer may experience through serious news, bereavement, terror, severe mental trauma, a feeling of desperation or a numbed, bemused state of mind. Every home should have a dropper bottle of it, and it's worth travelling with it. It is taken orally, at a dose of about 4 drops in water.

Homoeopathy

Homoeopathy is one of the more established of the complementary therapies but perhaps one of the least understood. As a broad medical approach it has much to offer, both in treating illness and helping in prevention of disease. It would appear that with skilled homoeopathic medication it is possible to treat an individual at a deep constitutional level, promoting health and wholeness on all levels.

In any approach to stress, anxiety, tension or other psychological 'dis-ease', it may well be that homoeopathy can hold the key to an individual's unique healing process. To use the homoeopathic remedies correctly and

effectively involves comprehending what is known as the 'symptoms picture'. It takes years of study and experience for a skilled homoeopathic to gain facility and ease with matching remedy to person.

It is impossible to talk of homoeopathic remedies for stress and anxiety. There are many specifics that might help but all depends upon the broader picture of physical health, general medical history, personality type, and so on.

No remedies will be recommended here and self-treatment with homoeopathic pills is to be avoided, but skilled homoeopathic treatment is of undoubted value and benefit. The important point is the skill, training and perception of the practitioner.

Diet

By now everyone has heard the expression 'You are what you eat'. Nowhere is this more true than in a person under stress and suffering from subsequent tension.

Ideally the food we eat and the way we eat it supplies us with all the nutrition we need and a time of relaxation in which to digest it. Most people are not ideal, however!

The normal diet of our society has been commented on so many times by everyone, from dieticians to the Government, that I shall focus on how to ensure that the nervous system is fed as well as the whole of body and mind. One point – avoid fad diets. They may be good for weight loss or whatever, but they are very bad for awareness and consciousness.

In general a healthy diet would be one rich in fresh, raw, green vegetables and fruit with a small amount of good meat if you can morally justify it to yourself. A major problem with meat in stress-related conditions is the feedstuff given to the animals, the chemicals that may have been used to stimulate growth, or whatever. Much of the current animal husbandry is straight out of a chemistry lab, something that we as consumers know little or nothing about. The diet should contain a fair proportion of roughage, but not buckets of bran! Wholemeal bread and a proportion of raw vegetables is fine.

A key to any dietary approach to health has to be the avoidance of artificial additives in any form. This will include flavours, colours and preservatives. Extremely difficult but vital.

A good supply of the vitamin B complex and vitamin C is essential. The C will come from fruit and most green vegetables, whilst the B is found in wholegrains, eggs, some fish, molasses and brewer's yeast.

There is much that should be avoided to help reduce anxiety and tension in general. As a priority there must be no food or drink containing caffeine as this adds to any agitation; this means coffee, tea and chocolate. Too much red meat can act as a physical stimulant and so might be avoided. Alcohol will be deleterious to the nervous system, amongst its other problems, and should be avoided, along with tobacco.

GENERAL INSTRUCTIONS

The way we eat affects the digestion of food. Eating should be a time of ease and peace. Here are some suggestions:

1 Small meals should be taken at regular intervals, every two or three hours if possible.
2 Eat your meals slowly and chew your food carefully.
3 Avoid rush and hurry before and after meals. Try to arrange a short rest before and after eating.
4 Sufficient sleep at night is important; aim at eight hours.
5 Remember that anxiety and worry can upset digestion.
6 Avoid large and heavy meals, fried food and anything that disagrees with you.
7 Never smoke or drink before meals.
8 Drink only sparingly during meals but take plenty of fluids *between* meals.

Body Work

The body holds the key for much of the strain that we carry around. Whole new areas of psychology are focusing on body/mind interactions, and as has already been hinted at, it is a mistake even to conceive body/emotion/mind as separate entities. We have seen how 'psychosomatic' illness can ground psychological anxieties in physical form as illness. In a similar way it is possible to relax the mind by easing the tension stored in the muscles of the body.

Many ways have been developed to do this and we shall discuss but a few. *Relaxation* techniques will be looked at in depth, followed by *yoga, dance, the Alexander Technique, Massage* and *Exercise* in general.

Relaxation

Perhaps the most important and simple of the tools we have for the reduction of the impact of stress is through the use of relaxation exercises.

When someone is tense and on edge, and has been so for a while, the worst thing to say is 'relax, take it easy'. That is guaranteed to put them even further on edge as they strain trying to relax!

Few of us today retain the innate skill of relaxation, a pity, but there it is. Relaxation is a skill that must be learnt and practised. There are vast ranges of relaxation techniques, some based on breathing, some on muscle control, some on visualization and some simply listening to music. It's a matter of finding what is most suitable for you.

Of the many varieties of relaxation exercises that we could explore, in this section we will focus on three: muscle awareness, rhythmic breathing and muscle contraction. Further relaxing techniques are described in the psychology section that follows. The first, muscle awareness, is examined more closely to show the general approach to doing this sort of thing.

MUSCLE AWARENESS

This technique, developed by Dr Harold Geld, is designed simply to develop your awareness of your larger muscles. It works most effectively if you let yourself be physically passive, but mentally aware and alert. It is the act of conscious attention that allows the muscles to relax.

Initially, it is best to practise this

awareness self-consciously at certain times, but then gradually it will become automatic, unconscious and continuous. Sometimes this muscle awareness is really all that's necessary in order for the brain's muscle-control centres to learn deep relaxation! Also, since muscles comprise a large portion of your body weight, learning to let them relax will lead to relaxation of your entire body.

For the first few times, perhaps have someone read the technique aloud to you, slowly, one sentence at a time, followed by 10–15-second pauses. Don't worry if you feel foolish and self-conscious. Why not?

By the third or fourth session, try doing the technique on your own, as best as you can remember it in your own mind. Don't be too concerned about precision, or remembering exactly every sequence of details. Instead, focus on adopting the correct general style.

In the earlier weeks of practising relaxation techniques, use common sense to avoid unnecessary distractions. For example:

1 Practise in a room alone, without any background radio or music.
2 Arrange to have someone answer the phone, if convenient, or take it off the hook during your practice.
3 Don't practice when you're in a hurry.
4 To avoid drowsiness, do not practice in the late evening or right after meals.

It seems a bit strange that I'm advising against drowsiness during a relaxation exercise. The point is not to slip into a sleep pattern but consciously, and with as much awareness as possible, to relax. If you do find yourself getting too

sleepy while practising a routine, then try one or more of the following:

1 Temporarily open your eyes, stretch your arms and take a couple of deep breaths; then resume the routine.
2 Practise during daylight, if possible.
3 Keep lights on bright instead of dim.
4 Practise in a sitting or semi-reclined position.
5 Vary the sequence of the muscle locations you focus on; for example, proceed from head to toe.
6 Shift your focus from one location to another more quickly than usual, and repeat the entire sequence a second time through.

Preparation for the technique

Lie down on your back, your heels several inches apart and your feet falling naturally to the sides. Let your arms lie out from your body at a comfortable angle, palms up or down – whatever's natural for you. Make any small adjustments in your hips, shoulders, neck and head until you feel as completely as possible 'sunk into the floor'.

With a few days' practice, you'll find this position more naturally and automatically comfortable. Use small pillows under your neck and lower back if necessary.

Now close your eyes and slowly take a couple of deep breaths. Begin to focus all your attention on how your breathing feels. Do not try to control the breathing pattern, but simply become aware of any or all of the following:

the rise and fall of the chest and stomach;
the slight stretching and loosening of some chest and rib-cage muscles with breath;

the small pause between each exhalation and inhalation;
the flow of air into the nose and throat (cool) and back out again (warm);
how far down into the lungs the air is flowing;
whether the depth of breathing seems uneven or regular;
any other physical sensations of the breathing process that you become sensitive to.

After a short time, your breathing will settle into a comfortable, steady, relaxed rhythm, and will no longer feel self-conscious, even though you are observing how it feels. It will seem to be a physical process that is happening naturally – that you're conscious of, but not interfering with. Continue this focus for another moment or so.

Now begin to focus on each of the muscle locations listed below. Do not move or contract the muscles in order to feel them better. Don't try to picture them in your mind. Don't recite this routine in your mind. Do not try to relax the muscles you're focusing on. Do not even 'try to feel' the muscles themselves. Simply direct your attention – focus all your awareness – into each location for a long, quiet moment. If there is any sensation to feel, you'll feel it without trying.

It does not matter what impression you get of each location as you come to focus on it (tense or relaxed, clear or vague or blank). It only maters that you quietly, effortlessly, focus on each place long enough (several breaths will usually do it) to become aware of it as a location, to become conscious of any slight or subtle feeling, if there's any at all.

Don't be concerned about mental distractions – for example, finding that your mind has wandered off to other thoughts. Distractions will always happen, so each time you become aware that you're distracted from the routine, simply return your attention to the point in the routine where you were last focusing.

The technique

1 Put your attention on your right and left calves. Imagine a point deep inside the centre of each calf muscle and become conscious of those two locations. Be aware of the pressure of their contact with the floor. The muscles may feel soft and sunk into the floor, or stiff and pressing against it. This will probably become as clear as it can ever be within the space of several breaths.

2 Now continue this style of awareness in the following locations – one pair of points, or one area, at a time – focusing deep inside the centre of each muscle:

arches of the feet
calves
middle of thighs
hips and buttocks
palms of the hands
thick upper portion of the forearms
middle of each upper arm
outside corner of each shoulder
stomach surface, or front abdominal muscles
chest surfaces and rib-cage (slightly stretching and loosening with the breathing)
lower back muscles (arched stiffly off the floor, or sunk down into it?)
upper back muscles (feel the press-

ure of contact with the floor),
base, back and sides of the neck
jaw hinges
cheeks
eyes
brow
temples
scalp

The awareness of some muscles can sometimes be very subtle, but be patient. Direct your attention to each of these locations in the outline every time you do the routine. Remember, it is not necessary to feel anything clearly in any given location, on any given day. It's only important to direct your attention to each location in its turn. It is the method that matters, not the 'results'. The value of this technique of awareness (rather than the results of each separate observation) will become clearer to you after you've been experiencing this routine for a couple of weeks. Meanwhile you will be surprised at how relaxed you become by the end of a practice session.

3 Now return your attention to your breathing. Become as fully aware of its sensations as you were at the beginning of the routine. In addition, become aware of the condition of your four limbs – whether they feel heavy, sinking into the floor; or light, floating, even missing completely; warm or cool, at the skin surface or deep inside; tight or loose, etc.

4 Become conscious of the entire length of your back, from the lower spine to the base of the neck. Be aware of whether your back feels generally stiff and pressing against the floor; or soft and sunk into the floor, as if melted into it. Become conscious of the surfaces of your

head and your facial features – the degree to which they feel blank, slack, drained, empty, expressionless, like a lifeless mask.

Now, for the next few moments plan on changing nothing at all – no stretching, no deep breathing, no shifting or fidgeting or any other voluntary movement. Leave everything exactly as it is, simply let your eyelids open so you can see the room above and around you.

At this moment you may feel a little disorientated. The room may seem 'dreamlike', or your body may feel 'unreal'. This is a typical (and harmless) reaction in the first week or two, especially when the practice has been a good one (clearly felt and deeply relaxing).

This moment of total physical passiveness but with the eyes open, sets a very important example for the brain. It demonstrates that you can think, hear, and even see, without the use of any muscles. It shows that you can be completely relaxed physically while mentally aware and attentive. After a week or so of practice, it will no longer feel strange to you.

Finally, when you feel like it, take a couple of deep breaths, slowly get up, and carry on.

OTHER RELAXATION EXERCISES
The general guidelines for approaching the two following exercises is the same as for that given in the muscle-awareness outline above.

RHYTHMIC ABDOMINAL BREATHING
Breathing is of great value in relaxation, particularly during the initial stages. The

person who is at ease with himself and his world breathes slowly, deeply and rhythmically. Breathing is the only automatic body function capable of conscious control and by controlling breathing it is possible to influence all autonomic and to a degree emotional responses.

When we are tense and anxious, our breathing pattern becomes shallower and faster, while when we are relaxed it is deeper, slower and more rhythmical. By practising breathing in this relaxed way it helps the mind and emotions to become calm and enable you to carry on. This very simple exercise can be done at home or even in the queue of the supermarket. Only you will know you are doing it once you become familiar with it.

Most of what is written here is self-evident but please bear with me!

Ideally this should be done twice a day for between five and fifteen minutes in a quiet room, free of disturbance.

Rest on your back with head and neck comfortably supported, with pillow under the knees to take the strain off them and the back.

Rest hands on upper abdomen, close your eyes and settle into a comfortable position.

Sitting in a reclining position may be better suited – try both positions.

Avoid distractions such as sunlight, a clock, animals, etc.

The aim is to breathe slowly, deeply and rhythmically. Inhalation should be slow, unforced and unhurried. Silently count to four, five or six. When inhalation is complete, let your chest naturally and slowly exhale through the nose. Count this breathing out, as when breathing in. *The exhalation should take as long as the inhalation.*

There should be no sense of strain. If initially you feel you have breathed your fullest at a count of three, that is all right. Gradually try to slow down the rhythm until a slow count of five or six is possible, with a pause of two or three between in and out breaths.

This pattern of breathing should be repeated fifteen to twenty times and since each cycle should take about fifteen seconds, this exercise should occupy a total of about five minutes.

Once the mechanics of this exercise have been mastered, introduce thoughts at different parts of the cycle. An example would be on inhalation try to sense a feeling of warmth and energy entering the body with the air. On exhalation, sense a feeling of sinking and settling deeper into the surface you are laying on.

On completion, do not get up immediately but rest for a minute or two, allowing the mind to become aware of any sensations of stillness, warmth, heaviness etc.

Once mastered, this exercise can be used in any tense situation with the certainty that it will defuse the normal agitated response and should result in a far greater ability to cope.

PROGRESSIVE MUSCULAR RELAXATION

Much psychological stress is stored in the large muscles of the body. This exercise is designed to release this store and so stop the messages of tension and stress going from muscle to brain. In this way the cycle of anxiety and tension can be broken. It is best to precede this exercise with a few cycles of deep breathing.

This differs from the first of the relaxation exercises in that it actively releases the tension rather than allowing the stored tension to ease its way from the body.

Either lay down or sit in a reclining chair.

Avoid distractions and wear clothes that do not constrict.

Starting with the *feet*, try to sense or feel that the muscles of the area are not actively tense.

Then deliberately tighten them, curling the toes under and holding the tension for five or ten seconds. Then tense the muscles *even more strongly*, for a further few seconds before letting all the tension go and sensing the wonderful feeling of release.

Try consciously to register what this feels like, especially in comparison with the tense state in which they were held.

Progress to the *calf* muscles and exercise in the same way. First sense the state the muscles are in, then tense them, hold the position, and then tense them even more before letting go. *Positively* register the sense of relief.

There is a slight possibility of inducing cramp doing this. If this occurs, stop tensing that area immediately and go on to the next.

After the calf go on to exercise the *knees*, then the *upper leg, thighs, buttocks, back, abdomen, chest, shoulders, arms, hands, neck, head and face.*

The precise sequence is irrelevant, as long as all these areas are 'treated' to the same process.

Some areas may need extra attention, for example in the abdomen. The tensing of these muscles can be achieved either by contracting (pulling in the tummy) or by stretching (pushing outwards). This variation in tensing is applicable to many muscles in the body.

There are between twenty and twenty-five of these 'areas', depending upon how you go about it. Each should be given at least 5–10 seconds of tensing and a further 5–10 seconds of letting go and passively sensing the feeling.

Thus 8–10 minutes should cover the whole technique. This should be followed by several minutes of an unhurried feeling of warm, relaxed tranquillity.

Focus the mind on the whole body. Sense it as heavy and content, free of tension or effort. This would be enhanced by a few cycles of deep breathing.

Have a good stretch and then carry on with your daily life.

Relaxation is a state of mind and body at ease and in poise; it is not a technique. If you do not find any of the three suggestions to your liking, fine. There are many others to try, but also different ways of approaching the body as a whole, which we shall now discuss.

Relaxation is about ease, so search ease out. This could be through some structured approach, such as yoga, jogging, enjoying dancing, etc. If it is appropriate in your life style, perhaps the most natural body mode for moving to poise and ease is sex. This is the most natural expression of human loving, caring attention that is expressed through the body.

Yoga

To do yoga justice involves years of commitment, practice and study. In

Britain, it has become freely available in the form of Hatha Yoga classes given by most local education authority evening classes. This is excellent and provides a way to enter a whole new world of stress management through body movement postures, breathing and relaxation.

It cannot be faulted as a form of body integration and exercise that relaxes and helps to bring about a sense of inner ease. In the religious and cultural atmosphere from which it stems this form of Hatha Yoga is but one step in a whole process of spiritual work and enlightenment. Maybe, one day soon, we will have classes in spiritual enlightenment in all further education centres!

I shall not give any suggestions as to positions (*asanas*) to use, as this should be done under the guidance of a good teacher, of which there are now many.

Dance

There is nothing new about humanity's love affair with dance, but it seems to be reaching new peaks of freedom and expression. Creative dance is a wonderful way to feel and express physical poise, which in turn is an expression of ease and relaxation. It is not the skill but the enjoyment that counts.

It doesn't matter whether we are talking about ballroom dancing, disco, ballet or break-dancing. What matters is the sense of release that often comes with this form of movement. There is a record by Will Powers called 'Dancing for Mental Health'! Dance with others, dance in formation, dance to music, dance through the woods . . .

Exercise

Any gentle exercise will have a toning effect on the body and will bring in its wake a sense of relaxation. For some more physical people this exercise is taken to the point of exhaustion. This goes beyond relaxation and can actually become a stress on the body.

Healthy exercise of any form should be part of a stress management programme, from gentle country walks all the way through jogging to hard-core aerobics. Choose what suits you. Be at ease with the process – that is always the clue to what is best.

Touch

Touching is one of the most natural human activities. We touch to comfort, to arouse, to communicate, and a whole range of therapeutic touch techniques have been developed. These range from gently rubbing a bruise to the skilled release of a lifetime accumulation of chronic tension in the muscles.

These touch-based approaches to healing work holistically in that they see mind/emotion and body working as one system. They acknowledge what we discussed earlier about the two-way flow from mind to body that can cause *psychosomatic* conditions and also the body-to-mind flow called *somatopsychic*. So working on the body with touch can ease the mind deeply.

Here we are concentrating on promoting greater relaxation, but there are touch-based therapies that are actively part of psychotherapeutic body work. Here the work of Reich and the field of bioenergetics are proving most useful. However, these fields go beyond the range of this book.

Massage

Massage is a beautiful way to relax. Of course the idea of massage embraces extremes from very physical and extreme manipulations given to rugby players to the sensual forms of gentle massage.

For relaxation it is always best to use the gentler forms that release body tension through skilled and caring movements. One of the most powerful things about massage is the very act of such intimate physical contact between two people. We don't touch much in our society, and when we do it has sexual connotations. Physical sensuality does not mean sexuality. It is an acknowledgement that the body deserves care and attention.

Massage should be used with the essential oils discussed in the section on aromatherapy. Here the double benefit of plant oils and human touch can achieve miracles.

In a book of this kind it is impossible to give a guide to massage for the whole body. There are a number of excellent guides to massage techniques that are simple to use and well illustrated. They are listed in the bibliography. Good masseurs are worth their weight in gold!

Shiatsu

Shiatsu is a very specialized form of massage, designed to relieve muscle tension and fatigue through direct pressure. Treatments consist of pressure on a specific sequence of points, designed to affect certain muscle systems. The basis for Shiatsu is in Chinese medicine which sees the roots of physical disease as energy imbalances in the major body systems of the body. One cause of energy blockage is muscular tension, and alleviating the tension brings back normal functioning.

The Alexander Technique

This is a way of becoming more aware of balance, poise and movement in every-day activities. This can bring into consciousness tensions previously unnoticed, and so help us differentiate between the tensions and efforts that are necessary for poise and those that aren't.

The Alexander Technique is concerned with posture and relaxation, two ideas not usually seen as one, and goes beyond relaxation as something one 'does', treating it instead as an attribute of being. There is a deep relationship between physical and psychological ease which can be seen at work in our posture.

Posture is far more complex than just sitting or standing straight. It can be described as how we support and balance our bodies against the ever-present pull of gravity whilst we go about our daily lives. There is a whole array of natural postural reflexes to organize this support and balance without any great effort, providing that we have the necessary degree of what has been called 'relaxation in activity' to allow these reflexes to work freely.

The mechanisms of support and balance, poise, are very delicate and are easily interfered with. The emotional and physical strains of life can soon become fixed in the body in the form of chronic muscle tensions and patterns of distortion throughout the body. Even our language expresses this knowledge – 'Things are getting me down' or 'I'm feeling uptight' both express well this relationship.

A teacher of the Alexander method uses gentle guidance with the hands to unravel the distortions and encourage reflexes to work again. In this way a balance can be found between the necessary degree of muscle tone (tension) needed to support the body against the pull of gravity, and the degree of relaxation to allow free movement, breathing, circulation and digestion.

In addition to manual methods, the teacher will give instruction to help the person become conscious of their own patterns of 'interference', suggesting ways to change these problems.

It is best to get skilled training and therapy, and advice on therapists can be obtained from: The Society of Teachers of the Alexander Technique, 10 London House, 266 Fulham Road, London SW10 9EL. In USA contact: The American Center for the Alexander Technique, 129 W 67th St, New York, NY10023 (212 799-0468).

Manipulation

The medical techniques of osteopathy and chiropractic may be helpful in releasing locked-in muscle tension or by relieving structural problems with the skeleton that cause muscular tension.

Such skilled work must only ever be undertaken by a skilled practitioner, in the hands of whom much can be achieved.

Mind and Emotions

Recent years have seen great advances made in the understanding of emotion and mind. Along the way have sprung up many approaches to enable us to recognize and heal the hurts and pains that accrue through life. We shall not look at them all, as this book deals primarily with the way in which herbs can help in stress and anxiety problems, but some of the useful insights are worth examining.

Any truly whole way of easing the impact of stress or soothing the anxieties of life must focus on our attitudes, expectations, assumptions and general perceptions of life. The way we feel is created by what has been called 'mind set'. This is the context of thoughts and beliefs that build up from the cradle to the grave, and is approachable and changeable. We can 'change our minds'.

All the ways that have been developed to enable psychological transformation to occur are worthy of a book on their own. In fact a whole library could be filled with the theories and techniques that have been developed.

In this section we shall briefly see what the role of psychological approaches can be, followed by some examples and self-help contacts.

Psychotherapy and Counselling

Psychotherapy is a range of procedures which involve the communication and relationship between client and therapist. This can take many forms, depending on the therapist's theoretical orientation, the client's problems and the aims of treatment. Despite the great range of approaches, the most universal characteristic is that all make use of an interpersonal situation in which the therapist communicates to the client that he or she understands, respects and wants to help.

Other features are the development of a rationale, or 'myth', explaining the distress and methods of dealing with it, exploring the source of the problem and exploring possible alternatives which hold a hope of relief. There is a boosting of self-esteem whilst facilitating the experience of success and of feeling good. Importantly it takes place in a locale designed as a place of healing.

A simple, but misleading, classification of procedures can be made into those which are essentially supportive in aim and those which seek to obtain a much deeper understanding of the person's past and present in order to bring about therapeutic changes. This subdivision is far from mutually exclusive. Insight therapies such as psychoanalysis or psychosynthesis may be very supportive for the person whilst a supportive relationship may help bring about insights and changes on the individual's part.

SUPPORTIVE PSYCHOTHERAPY

Supportive therapy is intended to offer support during a difficult period. In seeing a therapist at regular intervals during such a time, the person may be able to talk through fears and worries and in this way find a way of handling the difficulties. It is basically palliative and primarily intended to relieve distress. Regular contact with an accepting 'authority' figure and the opportunity to discuss problems, may lead to positive changes such as the restoration or strengthening of coping behaviours which may have been impaired by the stressful situation. The role of therapist is that of the accepting empathic listener, encouraging the person to talk, to express emotions and to help in dealing with guilt, shame or anxiety. Relatively little training may be necessary since the emphasis is more on listening than on skilful guidance or treatment.

It is of particular value when extreme stress gives rise to intense worry or anxiety and tends to be most effective when the client's personality is basically sound and the stressful situation is short-lived. Most medical herbalists as well as general practitioners would probably see this supportive role as one of their primary roles in our stressful times.

INSIGHT PSYCHOTHERAPIES

It is more difficult to summarize the aims and procedures associated with the interpretative methods. They are referred to as 'insight' or 'reconstructive' therapies since they are concerned with giving the patient increased self-understanding and bringing about changes in attitudes, goals and emotional responses. They range from the analytical approach of classical psychoanalysis to newer therapies based on a spiritually integrated view of what humanity may be. Such therapies must be used by skilled practitioners and involve a degree of commitment and motivation on the part of the client.

This is not the right place to go into this in depth, but holistic insight psychotherapy can in the right time and place enable changes to occur that completely transform the people involved.

Contact can be made with counsellors and psychotherapists either through a medical practitioner or by finding one yourself. The address list of self-help groups given at the end of this chapter will guide you – The British Association for Counselling, 1a Little Church Street, Rugby, Warwickshire CV21 3AP, (0788 78328) is particularly helpful.

Autogenic Training

This therapy is growing in use and acceptance by orthodox medicine in Britain, with many hospitals providing AT clinics and classes. A welcome sign! Whilst this is a relaxation therapy, it works through psychological pathways and so is included in this section. It could for other reasons have been in the section on body work.

Autogenic training (AT) is a highly systematized technique designed to generate a state of 'psychophysiologic relaxation' – a state completely physically opposite to that occurring under stress. Through the generation of this state, termed the autogenic (self-generated) state, the recuperative and self-healing processes of the person are brought into play, presumably through effects on the autonomic nervous system. This technique forms the foundation for the more inclusive system known as autogenic therapy.

THE STANDARD EXERCISES

Six standard exercises form the foundation of autogenic training. These exercises are taught in a very structured fashion. Following the completion of a detailed medical/psychological history, the individual is instructed in a specific training posture (intended to reduce to a mimimum any distracting stimuli), the proper way to end the exercises, and the phrases themselves. The individual then practises these techniques for several minutes at least three times a day and keeps a log of his or her experiences. The

trainer monitors the trainee's progress and determines from observations of the trainee and his or her reports from the training sessions and from home practice (log entries) whether the trainee is ready to move on to the next exercise.

Each exercise involves the use of a specified phrase intended to generate a particular physiological state. While practising, the trainee is instructed to 'attend' passively to a particular body part while mentally repeating one of the phrases. For example, the first exercise is concerned with the generation of heaviness in the extremities. The trainee begins by passively attending to his dominant arm and mentally repeating a number of times 'my right (left) arm is heavy'. Following the focus on this arm, he or she is then encouraged to generalize the heaviness to all limbs (i.e. 'My left (right) arm is heavy'; 'Both arms are heavy'; 'My arms and legs are heavy') before moving on to the next exercises. The exercises are summarized in Table 3.

Table 3: The six standard autogenic training exercises

Standard exercise	Physiological state	Phrase
1	Heaviness in the extremities	'My arms and legs are heavy.'
2	Warmth in the extremities	'My arms and legs are warm.'
3	Calm and regular function of the heart	'My heart is calm and regular.'
4	Calm and regular breathing	'My breath is calm and regular.'
5	Solar plexus warm	'My solar plexus is warm.'
6	Forehead cool	'My forehead is cool.'

ADJUNCTIVE TECHNIQUES

There are four, so called adjunctive techniques of AT, which are: autogenic modification, autogenic neutralization, autogenic meditation, and interdisciplin-

ary techniques. We shall look at the first three:

1 *Autogenic modification* uses the autogenic state as a way of bringing about specific changes. This approach in-

volves a phrase, used in addition to or in combination with the standard exercises, that focuses either on physiological change or an attitudinal/behavioural change. Using an organ-specific formula, a trainee with chronic constipation adds the phrase, 'My lower abdomen is warm' to the standard exercises in order to stimulate movement of the bowels. The use of 'Breath carries the words' by a stutterer, and 'I am satiated' by an obese individual, are other examples of intentional formulas.

2   *Autogenic neutralization* allows the carefully supported release of feelings in order to neutralize or reduce their disturbing effects. The trainee is encouraged to talk about either material related to a theme or whatever comes to mind. Of crucial importance in the practice of these techniques is the maintenance of an attitude of passive acceptance by both trainee and trainer – an attitude of neither suppressing nor enhancing the sensations, just allowing the sensations to be while continuing AT.

3   *Autogenic meditation* consists of a series of seven exercises begun only after the trainee has developed the ability to maintain passive concentration for at least thirty minutes (usually after at least six months of AT practice). The focus of the exercises progresses from colour, concrete objects and images, feelings, and persons to a state where the trainee directly poses questions to the unconscious.

Process of Desensitization

Relaxation is all very well for those rare times of peace and quiet when you can go through the techniques outlined. It is possible, however, to use similar approaches to desensitize or dis-identify with a particularly problematic situation. In other words actually change the way you react to the world. Much good counselling aims at this, but there is a simple way to start the process yourself.

A good first step is to take a sheet of paper, sit down for a few minutes, and write out a list of people, places, activities and circumstances that you know produce tension in you. You should include only those items which come up regularly in your daily or weekly life. Some possible examples could include:

dealing with your spouse

dealing with an in-law

dealing with your own parents

dealing with your own children

dealing with any children (a good one for teachers!)

dealing with or just facing your boss

meeting deadlines

making an important decision

giving speeches or oral reports

taking a test or exam

competing, at work or games

driving in heavy traffic

driving long distances

being in a crowded room

being in a very small space

being in a very wide open space

looking down from a height

waking up/ getting up in the morning

visting a doctor

visiting a dentist

taking pills

cooking, cleaning or other housework

typing or other desk work (writing a book!)

working out your tax return

being in a lift   any other person, place, activity or situation.

Include in your list only those things that cause a distinct physical tension or anxiety response in you. Some may be very strong but others may be a lot milder in their effects on you. But they all should be things that come up regularly or periodically.

Keep this list with you, and for the next week or so, when you notice yourself tensing up over anything at all, make sure you add that cause to your list. As soon as your list has at least a half-dozen entries, you can begin the process of desensitization, by which you should learn to be at ease with those very things that used to get you tense.

In order for it to work well for you, you must follow it consistently for a few weeks, but without impatiently expecting dramatic results. Remember, your stress reactions have developed and become ingrained in you over a long period of time. A lot of your physical tension is an unconscious habit by now. This is not reversible overnight. As in learning any skill – or unlearning any bad habit – it takes a while to create or undo behaviour patterns, and you will do so only by consistent practice.

First look at the list. Choose an item that is moderate in its effect on you (not your strongest tension producer, and not the weakest). Let it be something that comes up pretty often, say more than once a week. An additional advantage would be if it's something that occurs at specific, predictable times. This makes it much easier to prepare for, with the appropriate training steps we will discuss below.

It doesn't matter what the trigger of the tension is. You can learn to be at ease in this recurring situation by following these steps:

1   After doing a full relaxation exercise, when feeling deeply relaxed, start to imagine clearly the situation that causes you distress. Visualize in as much depth and clarity as possible, the physical situation and people involved. Start at the beginning of the situation and run through in your imagination the series of events as they would normally occur.

You should envision the whole sequence as clearly and realistically as possible, seeing and hearing everything as you would in 'real life'. If at any time in the exercise you actually respond with muscular tension or breathing changes, then stop for a moment. Instead, focus on your breathing and be aware of your muscles, allowing yourself to sink back into a relaxed state again. Only then continue the imagining where you left off. Each time you feel any physical tension at all, let go of the fantasy, regain the calm state and breathe into it deeper with each exhalation.

2   The next step is to use your awareness when out in the world but *not* in the particular situation you fantasized. Take a few moments and do some of the breathing exercises described above. This will enable you to relax into an easy poise. Imagine the situation in your mind whilst feeling this poise.

3   Do this exercise and the breathing more often as the particularly problematic situation approaches. This builds up to prepare and desensitize you to the trauma you have planted

inherently in the situation. This is designed to train your body to remain relaxed in those very situations you would usually brace yourself for. You can learn to be mentally responsible and concerned without having to suffer the physical symptoms.

After a week or so the first target of desensitization will be causing you less tension. Next choose another on your list and do the same process all over again around it. You will find that each new target gets easier and quicker to relax into. Not only will you learn to deal with specific situations, you'll have acquired a general skill of being physically relaxed as a habit.

Most importantly, enjoy yourself as you become calmer and more in control of your life and its reactions.

Social Support

Many of the stresses that assail us are compounded by our helplessness in the face of problems. Maybe once people were able to cope with anything that came their way, but today life has become far too complex. These complexities can become almost insurmountable when we feel helpless and isolated with not one to turn to. It is in these times that turning to others can be so important. They can, of course, provide useful advice, but much more important is the experience of shared human feeling and understanding that can be found.

We are not concerned here with the excellent but rather cumbersome official agencies, but the growing number of self-help and support groups now in existence. They are a wonderful expression of the care and compassion that people show for each other when the need arises.

However, do not forget the help that is offered by the Welfare State in all its forms. Whilst the system is a problem, it is filled and run by caring and skilled people. The social services departments, health centres, etc. are there to provide help and support.

A selection of self-help groups, with addresses and a brief description of their work, is given below. It is not a comprehensive list but provides a place to start. If a group or agency that would be able to help you is not listed here, contact your local Citizen's Advice Bureau.

National Marriage Guidance Council
Herbert Gray College, Little Church Street, Rugby, Warwickshire CV21 3AP (0788 73241)
A wonderful organization of well-trained but voluntary counsellors. They provide help and guidance in all aspects of the problems that arise in married life. The local address can be found in the telephone directory under 'Marriage Guidance Council'.

Scottish Marriage Guidance Council
26 Frederick Street, Edinburgh EH2 2JR (031-225 5006)

Catholic Marriage Guidance Council
15 Lansdowne Road, London W11 3AJ (01-727 0141)

Jewish Marriage Council
23 Ravenshurst Avenue, London NW4 4EL (01-203 6311)

American Association for Marriage and Family Therapy
1717 K St, Suite 407, Washington DC 20006, USA (202 429-1825)

Gingerbread
35 Wellington Street, London WC2
(01-240 0953)
Nationwide organization that provides
support for single parents and their
children. There are self-help groups
throughout the country and a phone-in
advice service each weekday afternoon.

National Council for One-Parent Families
255 Kentish Town Road, London NW5
2LX (01-267 1361)
Offers help, advice and counselling. The
service is free and confidential, including
legal advice and help with problems such
as housing, social security, taxation and
maintenance.

Parents Without Partners
7910 Woodmont Ave, Suite 108, Bethesda, MD 20814, USA (301 654-8850)

National Council for the Divorced and Separated
13 High Street, Little Shelford, Cambridge CB2 5ES (0206 396206)

National Federation of Solo Clubs for Widowed, Divorced, Separated and Single People
7/8 Ruskin Chambers, 191 Corporation Street, Birmingham 4 (021-236 2879)

CRUSE, National Organization for the Widowed and Their Children
126 Sheen Road, Richmond, Surrey
(01-940 4818)
Provides a counselling service to widows
and widowers, practical advice and
opportunities for social contact.

The Compassionate Friends
2 Norden Road, Blandford, Dorset
DT11 7LT (0258 52760)
An organization of bereaved parents
who seek to help other bereaved parents
by giving them the opportunity to speak
freely to an understanding and compassionate friend.

The Compassionate Friends
PO Box 1347, Oak Brook, Illinois
60521, USA (312 323-5010)

Depressives Anonymous
Self-Help Centre, 83 Derby Road, Nottingham NG1 5BB

Depressives Associated
19 Merley Way, Wimborne Minster,
Dorset (0202 883957)
A self-help service for depressives, run
by ex-sufferers who have a direct understanding of the problems of depression.

The Samaritans
170 local branches – look in telephone
directory.

Samaritans USA
PO Box 480, Falmouth, Mass 02540 (617
548-8900)

Women's Aid Federation
374 Grays Inn Road, London WC1
(01-837 9316)
Aims to assist physically and mentally
battered women. There are groups
throughout the country.

Scottish Women's Aid
11 St Colme Street, Edinburgh (031-225
8011)

Welsh Women's Aid
2 Coburn Street, Cardiff (0222 388291)

Family Network (01-226 2033)
A phone-in service run by the National
Children's Home to assist with problems
such as family violence, battering of
wives, child abuse, drugs. It operates in
most areas and is usually advertised on
local radio, newspapers, etc.

National Organization for Women
1401 New York Ave, NW, Washington
DC 20005-2102, USA (202 347 2279)

Organization for Parents under Stress
Information Offices, 26 Manor Drive,
Pickering, N. Yorks YO18 8DD (0602
470551)
A co-ordinating body under the umbrella name of OPUS that can give parents
the phone number of a group in their
part of the country.

Parents Anonymous Inc
22330 Harthorne Blvd 208, Torrance,
CA 90505
(213 371-3501)

British Association for Counselling
1a Little Church Street, Rugby, Warwickshire CV21 3AP (0788 78328)
Will put people in touch with a counselling service or with individual counsellors
who are members of the association.

Action on Smoking and Health (ASH)
Margaret Pyke House, 27-35 Mortimer
Street, London W1 (01-637 9843)
Issues free leaflets and lists of local
authority smoking withdrawal clinics.

Alcoholics Anonymous
PO Box 514, 11 Redcliffe Gardens,
London SW10 9BG (01-352 9779)
468 Park Ave S, New York, NY 10016,
USA (212 686-1100)
A world-wide voluntary fellowship of
people whose aim, mutually reinforced,
is to attain and maintain sobriety. There
are no fees, the only desire for membership is the desire to stop drinking.
The programme is one of total abstinence, based on staying away from drink
one day at a time. The local AA number
can be found in the local telephone
directory.

Al-Anon
Family Groups, 61 Great Dover Street,
London SE1 4YF (01-403 0888)
1372 Broadway, New York, NY 10018,
USA (212 302-7240)
Helps relatives and friends of problem
drinkers, whether or not the drinker
seeks help or even recognizes the need to
do so. Anonymity is strictly preserved.

Standing Conference on Drug Abuse
(SCODA)
3 Blackburn Road, London NW6 1XA
(01-328 6556)
An umbrella organization for the different voluntary bodies concerned with
drug misuse and can refer people to
sources of personal advice and counselling.

Narcotics Anonymous
PO Box 622, Sun Valley, CA 91352,
USA (213 764-4880)

Release
1 Elgin Avenue, London W9 3PR
(01-289 1123)
Assists with information on drugs and
the law relating to drugs, and with
referrals for treatment. They can advise
on problems with tranquillizers.

Spiritual Integration

All the ways towards a state of inner ease so far discussed have been to do with the outer world and our relationship with it. Herbs seen as gifts of our world to ease our path through life; massage and relaxation as ways of soothing a tense and troubled body; counselling to ease the storm of emotions that tends to drown us at times. There is another way to approach all of this, a way that starts from within the human psyche, at its very core.

There is a spiritual, ineffable centre to all human life and to all motivation and action. This spiritual centre, whether we call it the soul, the life force or whatever, is the source of our individual lives; it is the light that illuminates and source of inner healing and ease. It is Well-Being.

There are many ways to approach the spirit. Of course, religion is, in theory, the path of approach, but in these times of chaos some of the religious structures evolved over the years have become somewhat limiting in themselves. For a committed Christian, Jew, Moslem, Buddhist, etc., there is open to them a door through which meaning, spiritual love and, indeed, God are reachable. It is an openness and a real alignment with things spiritual that is the core of all real ease. We could say God is the best remedy for stress!

The spirit is freely available to all, no matter what beliefs are held. Religion is but one way, and it is within the reach of us all to find this centre. It is from here that peace and joy flow into our lives, and so why not turn there to experience the 'peace that passeth all understanding'?

Meditation and other ways of inner stilling do not compromise one's beliefs. A Christian can meditate without it being a denial of the creed, a Jew can meditate without it being a denial of his faith. In the West, meditation has an Eastern 'occult' aura about it which is completely ridiculous and unfounded. In this section of the book meditation will be considered practically as a way to ease tension and achieve some inner poise. However, that is but a first stage in the meditative process, going deeper is beyond this book but not beyond you.

Love and Meaning

Many people today are profoundly uneasy with their lives and the direction in which our whole society is moving.

This unease is often too deep to be felt for what it is or too uncomfortable to be spoken of. However, it is an increasingly shared experience. We have not only become separated from our roots in planet Earth, alienated from our fellows, but most dangerously, there seems to be a split in our awareness of our own selves. The love that is a keynote of being human and the purpose and vision that give our lives meaning seem to have been lost. Our myths and legends talk of a golden age, when in truth the golden age is in our own heart and soul here and now.

The all-pervasive atmosphere of alienation and separation takes some obvious forms. There is the ecocrisis, economic collapse, world-wide starvation whilst grain mountains fill Europe, all enveloped in the fear of nuclear megadeath. These massive issues may seem out of the hands of us simple folk, but there is a direct relationship between such a situation and, for example, the personalized stresses that cause migraine. It can be argued that much stress-related physical illness is the whole human malaise taking individual form. We could say that humanity as a whole has migraine at the moment!

This is not meant to put the weight of planetary ills on each of our shoulders, but to show that there is more going on than we think or feel. A way for each of us to start is to clear up the 'ecocrisis' in our lives, to get rid of the emotional and spiritual starvation we often consider to be normality. We can change the world and we can change ourselves.

The only permanent 'cure' for anxiety, tension and depression is an experience of the solid foundations and soaring potential of who we are. The wisdom of love, and the hope that springs from vision, heals and brings inner ease. Not always outer ease, for the insights gained will often prompt much activity in the world, but within is an inner stance of poise that is a healing well-spring of peace.

Prayer

A profound and wonderful way of achieving inner peace is through the path of prayer. Prayer is a way of communing, or approaching, with the spirit. It doesn't really matter what you call this spiritual centre of love and wisdom, whether it be God, Christ or one's own inner self, the reality of its healing presence remains the same. All spiritual paths have their own ways of prayer, each individual develops his or her own way of praying.

It is worth noting that in English the word for prayer and the person praying – the prayer – are the same. There is a hint here that in a deep and mysterious way we become the path, we become the prayer as we use it.

In this book we shall not be suggesting specific prayers to use or ways to do it, rather simply reminding you that inner ease is a gift which comes with selfless prayer.

Meditation

Whenever someone concentrates and focuses their attention, they are meditating. This could be a 'captain of industry', someone planting a herbaceous border or a Zen monk. The difference is the degree to which they are focusing and the purpose of the whole exercise.

Meditation can be a profound and powerful tool in the expansion of consciousness and an exploration of spirit; however, it is just as relevant as a gentle way of moving to a place of ease and poise within. The term meditation covers a whole spectrum of approaches and techniques, but here we shall concentrate on simple aids in the reduction of stress and the nurturing of inner ease. In the West, in these days of crisis and transformation, we are fortunate indeed to have increasingly much of the spiritual wisdom and skill of the East available to us. A plethora of teachers, schools and books is ready to help in exploring the more profound depths of meditation. The techniques described below may whet your appetite for a deeper plunge. Don't hesitate! Much of the stress and strain of existence has its roots in a lack of meaning, a sense of unfulfilment in what we do and why we do it. Meditation can point they way to the source of inner meaning, if you want it to.

LEVELS OF MEDITATION
Western medical research has focused upon meditation as a way to gain control, a 'self-regulation strategy'. This research was initially interested in the physiological changes that occur during meditation. Certain changes have been consistently reported during meditation, including a reduction in heart rate, a decrease in bodily oxygen consumption, a lowering of blood pressure, an increase in skin resistance, and an increase in the regularity and strength of alpha activity in the brain. Because this represents a state of quietness in the autonomic nervous system, doctors suggested that meditation would be a useful self-regulation technique for relaxation training.

Unsurprisingly, the clinical research has borne this out. In a recent academic review of the psychotherapeutic and health-related effects of meditation its value was shown in:

1 Reducing stress and tension where meditators show both subjective reports of decreased feelings of stress and anxiety as well as objective physiological indications of stress reduction.
2 Decreasing addictive behaviours. In studies of addictions meditators consistently report a larger reduction in usage than non-meditators for drugs ranging from alcohol and marijuana to LSD and heroin.
3 Lowering blood pressure. The research consistently shows a reduction in blood pressure in meditators, a reduction in the use of medication, and a reduction of bodily symptoms.

This scientific appraisal of meditation also shows how the therapist is changed by the process of healing or helping. Reports from therapists using meditation in their work report that it helps them become more open and receptive to their clients' concerns.

MEDITATION AS AN ALTERED STATE OF CONSCIOUSNESS
Most research in the West has been carried out in laboratories and settings with relatively short-term meditators. Remember, however, that meditation was originally conceived within a philosophical–religious context of the Eastern spiritual disciplines. It was a technique used primarily as a means for inducing altered states of consciousness, for changing a person's ordinary perception of the world, and for developing a more intimate, unified, and accepting view of oneself, of nature, and of other people.

There can be no doubt that when used in this way profound changes can occur during meditation. These can range from slight alterations in perception in short-term meditators to more profound experiences. The following descriptions from meditators may give a taste of the possibilities: 'self-transcendence'; 'felt meaning in the world'; 'a heightened sense of connectedness with the world and with others, a sense of purpose and meaningfulness, deep positive emotion'.

These very powerful inner experiences have obvious implications for health because they influence the way we relate not only to ourselves but also to other people and to the world around us. Just as important are the social implications, as people who use meditation in this way transform themselves and their approach to life. It is one of the signs of hope for the future that a growing number of people meditate and are willing to put into practice the re-appraisal it brings about.

TECHNIQUES

There are hundreds of practices which could be called meditation. The devices used to bring about the meditative state are as diverse as gazing quietly at a candle flame, concentrating on the mental repetition of a sound or *mantra*, following one's own breathing, concentrating on the imagined sound of rainfall, chanting out loud a ritual word or phrase, attending to body sensations, passively witnessing the flow of thoughts through the mind, concentrating on an unanswerable riddle, or whirling in a dance.

The aim is always the same – to alter the way the meditator experiences his or her own existence. What follows is a simple guide to basic types of meditation and how to use them in practice.

PREPARATION FOR MEDITATION

Meditation will only be effective in stress reduction or spiritual development if one is properly prepared and in a receptive frame of mind. Here are some suggestions for such preparation. You will notice the similarities to the guidelines for approaching relaxation and sleep.

1 Don't meditate within an hour after having a meal. The meditative traditions insist that meditation is ineffective on a full stomach. Coffee, tea and caffeine-containing drinks such as *Coca-Cola* should be avoided. The need to avoid stimulants should be obvious – meditation is for calming down.

2 Choose a quiet room to meditate in, where you can be alone. If someone else is present he or she should be meditating as well. Take the phone off the hook or cover it with a thick pillow. Let others in the house know you are meditating and that you would apreciate stillness. Don't have any pets around in case they disturb you. It can be quite a shock to have a cat jump on your lap when in meditation!

3 Face away from any direct light, and whilst the room need not be dark it is more pleasant if the lighting is subdued.

4 Sit in a comfortable, easy position. This could be a straight-backed chair or a cushion on the floor. It will help to loosen tight clothes and remove shoes. It is best to have your back straight.

5 If during meditation you become uncomfortable, change your position slightly, stretch, yawn or scratch. When using meditation for stress

reduction, the point is to be at ease and is not an exercise in the discipline of a Zen monk. Such disciplines focus on mastering distractions and not necessarily being at ease.

6 If you are interrupted try not to jump up out of meditation suddenly. You are likely to be in a deeply relaxed state, so gently and slowly stretch and then get up. Ideally return to meditation afterwards.

7 The length of a meditation session is up to you. Times are suggested for each technique, but may not feel comfortable initially. Take as long or as short as feels comfortable.

8 If you find that meditation suits you, schedule sessions into your life so as to make them a regular daily routine. Occasional use of the technique, while pleasant, will not bring about any lasting benefits. It is best to meditate twice a day but you should try to do so at least once daily.

9 After finishing, remain seated for a moment or two with your eyes closed. During this time allow your mind to return to everyday thoughts. This helps to carry the tranquillity into your daily life. Then, very slowly, open your eyes and get up leisurely.

ATTITUDE

The techniques described below should not prove difficult even for those unfamiliar with meditation. They should be approached with a gentle, non-forcing attitude. It is best to try not to do the meditation exercises 'correctly', but to let each meditation 'do' itself. There is no 'good' and 'bad' here.

Meditating to aid stress reduction does not involve focusing the mind. When-

ever thoughts enter (and they will often) simply treat them as you might clouds drifting across the sky. Don't try to push them away or hold on to them, simply watch them come and go. When you realize that your mind is caught up in thoughts, gently come back to your object of focus without forcing. The extraneous thoughts are a natural part of the meditative process.

MANTRA MEDITATION

Mantra or sound meditation is based on using a word or syllable as a focus for concentration. Select one of the three mantras suggested below, or use a word of your own choosing. Avoid using a word that is emotionally 'loaded'. No names of people, no words that bring too intense or exciting an image. It should ring in your mind and bring a sense of serenity. If you tell someone close to you the mantra you have chosen ensure they understand that regardless of their response to it, your mantra is to be respected. It will come to have a special meaning for you and will become a signal to turn inward towards a peaceful state.

When choosing your mantra. first repeat each of the suggestions (either mentally or out loud) and then select the one that sounds the most pleasant and soothing. The first two are traditional Indian mantras. Use one of your own choosing if you like.

Mantras: Ah-nam
Ra-ma
Peace (etc.)

Having selected your mantra, sit down comfortably.

With your eyes open and resting on a pleasant object such as a plant, say

61

the mantra out loud to yourself, repeating it slowly and rhythmically.

Experiment with the sound, play with it.

As you repeat it, say it softer and softer, until finally it becomes a whisper.

Stop saying it out loud, close your eyes, and simply listen to the mantra in your mind.

Let your facial muscles relax and think the mantra but do not say it.

That is all there is to meditating – sitting peacefully, hearing the mantra in your mind, allowing it to change any way it wants – to get louder or softer; to disappear or return; to stretch out or to speed up. Meditation is like drifting on a stream in a boat without oars – you don't need oars because you are not going anywhere.

Continue meditating for fifteen minutes. When the time is up, just sit quietly without meditating for another 2–3 minutes.

MEDITATING ON THE BREATH

There are some ancient and powerful techniques based on breath. These are not primarily for helping with relaxation but for personal and spiritual transformation. The guidelines here are very basic and aid the relaxation process.

Sit in a comfortable position and take a single slow deep breath, thinking to yourself the word 'In' as you breathe in, and the word 'Out' as you breathe out.

After taking this first deep breath, do not intentionally influence your breathing.

Let your breathing go its own way, fast or slow, shallow or deep, whatever way it wishes.

As it does so think to yourself 'In' on every in breath and 'Out' on every out breath.

After a while try to extend the sound in your mind so that at all points in the meditation you are either thinking 'In . . .n . . .n . . .' or 'Ouuuuuuut . . . t . . . t' in long, easy sounds.

Do this meditation naturally, with no concern about its correctness. If you skip an 'In' or 'Out' because your mind has wandered (as it will), you can always pick up the words on the next breath whenever you are ready.

If the words fade and you are just sensing the breath, that's fine and means you have quieted down.

When fifteen minutes are up, come out of meditation gradually and gently.

VISUAL MEDITATION

Select a pleasant natural object such as a plant, flower, piece of fruit, bit of driftwood, or some simple vase. Although a candle flame is sometimes used for visual meditation, it is not suggested here because its glare may cause eye strain if not properly used.

Place your chosen object on a table at or near eye level and at a distance of two to four feet from you. Adjust this distance according to the most comfortable focus for your own eyes and eliminate distracting objects in the immediate background.

Sit comfortably and allow your eyes to come to rest on the object, but do not try to see it. Make no effort to focus. Instead, allow the object to come into your vision – let it enter your awareness.

Do not make any conscious

attempt to think about it in any way – what it is, what it means, its name, the class of objects it belongs to, although if such thoughts come to your mind spontaneously, that is fine. Just look at your object innocently as a child might.

Avoid staring at any time, for this can cause eye strain. During this meditation your eyes will spontaneously want to move about, travel over the object. Allow them to do this. Do not stop your eye movements – this is part of 'seeing'.

Because most of us can only look at things with 'the eye of the beginner' for a few seconds at a time (unless highly trained) this meditation consists of a series of new beginnings.

After allowing the object to remain in your field of vision for about 7–10 seconds (this interval may be longer or shorter according to your own inclinations), purposely shift your eyes to a more distant place in the room. At this time you can remove your mental attention from the object as well, and let it wander where it will.

Continue repeating this process – gazing away from the object for a few seconds (you will 'feel' the right length for this time interval) and then, when you are ready, bringing your eyes and your attention back to it easily. Each time simply allow yourself to become absorbed in the object once more (again for about 7–10 seconds) and then systematically remove your gaze once again.

Continue in this way – looking at the object, looking away from it, and then returning to it refreshed – for five minutes (this is a shorter meditation than the other forms). At the end of five minutes close your eyes for a

minute or so and sit quietly.

This gives a range of simple meditation techniques to try out. If you feel at home with them you may wish to go further and deeper, in which case it is always best to find a teacher of meditation to help you.

Spiritual Healing

The spirit acts directly upon us but also can be 'directed' or invoked by a spiritual healer. As a book on herbal medicine for anxiety and stress, this is not the place to explore this deep and profound realm. However, there is much excellent work done by spiritual healers. Whilst many are 'non-professionals', there is a federation of healers in Britain whose address is: National Federation of Spiritual Healers, Old Manor Farm Studio, Church Street, Sunbury-on-Thames, Middlesex TW16 6RG.

A basic duty of the Ministry of the Church is healing the sick. Not all of our priests feel at ease with this work, but at times of stress and when anxieties abound, the Church can be a haven of peace.

Herbs and Spiritual Peace

It is completely natural for a herbalist to be at home in matters spiritual. One of the ways in which joy enters our hearts is through the beauty of nature and especially of the wild flowers. This is no coincidence. As much as plant remedies are potent internal medicines, they are also vital for a healthy world. No human being can remain sane for too long if deprived of plants and natural surroundings. Why do people fill their offices with indoor plants? Of course, because they are aesthetic, and I would suggest that it is through the subtler sensibilities that spirituality maintains our sanity.

A walk amongst the hedgerows, woods and meadows in the spring is a wonderfully healing thing to do. Why shouldn't we love our plants and even talk to them; there is no doubt that they love us!

The Bach flower remedies are an example of a direct link between plants as medicine and plants as spiritual agents.

Consider the humble cordial, a fruity non-alcoholic drink. It has its origins in the use of Borage flowers to make a drink that uplifted, eased depression and warmed the heart. Cordial comes from the Latin word for heart, Cor. To the medieval monks it was obvious and practical that God, through the simple flowers of the field, had given humanity a gift of healing and peace. Today we are at last relearning this simple truth

Throughout this book I have tried, where appropriate, to show the ways in which herbal remedies link us to our spiritual selves through our beloved planet, Earth. This connection with the foundation of the earth aligns us with yet greater realms of spirit and light. We are indeed one with the Creator of all things.

Let us use our herbal remedies with thankfulness and joy, for their very existence is a demonstration of God's unbounding love for us all.

Stress and Illness

When a person is seen as a whole individual – and not simply a body that has a mind on top of it, it comes as no surprise to realize that there is a deep association between both psychology and physiology. This has profound implications in all illness and not just in anxiety and depression.

The complex and diverse ways in which mind and body interact are wonderful indeed and only slightly understood or even perceived. It is a demonstration of the inadequacies of our scientific approach to this question that it is even phrased in terms of a separation of mind and body. As has already been discussed, they are in reality one system that should not be separated. However, to do this in the medium of English and say what needs to be said here, is exceedingly difficult!

It is worth examining how orthodox medicine sees the relationship between mind, body and spirit in the development of illness. Whilst no all-encompassing explanation for the association in disease has been put forward, there are a number of possible explanations:

1 Some physical illness may be psychological in origin; that is, the bodily disturbance is the result of and caused by the psychological illness.
2 Physical illness may arise as an indirect consequence of any mental disorder, the bodily illness resulting from behavioural disturbances which are secondary to the psychiatric problem.
3 Physical methods of treatment of mental illness may cause bodily disease. This is unfortunately all too common with the wide use of drug therapy today.
4 The mental disturbance may be a manifestation of any physical illness present, or an adverse effect of its treatment.
5 A mental or emotional problem may be a 'purely' psychological response to the illness or the significance that illness has for the person involved.

This might all sound a bit of a quibble! It is, however, a way of fitting the relationship of mind and body into a pattern that will then enable an orthodox medical practitioner to decide which drugs to use. Should he or she focus on the physical problems or the mental disturbance?

From the perspective of a holistic herbalist this is an artificial and unnecessary question. To help both body and mind the whole must be treated as a whole. Thus, not only remedies that may be helpful for emotional or digestive symptoms, but a management plan to help the person cope with the stress, is necessary. This broader view will lessen the impact of the stress, help free the person involved and hopefully create the space for healing to take place.

Emotional and Mental Responses to Physical Illness

Any illness occurs within the context of the person's whole life and so will effect the individual psychologically and socially as well as bodily. It is worth considering ways in which illness itself may produce psychological problems. The difference between this and a problem that affects the body but arises in the mind is purely one of perspective. Technically, if the doctor considers the primary problem to be in the mind it will be called a *psychosomatic* problem, but if the root is in the body it will be called *somatopsychic*:

psyche——(psychosomatic)——disease
disease——(somatopsychic)——psyche

Psychological reactions to physical illness are common and may need some sort of specialized help. This may be an orthodox psychiatrist, a more holistic health practitioner or simply talking to a friend.

The ignorance about psychological responses to physical illness found in most health practitioners reflects a narrow view of the nature of illness. When the 'illness' is seen in strictly biological terms it ignores the *patient's* own reality of the problem. For the patient there is no difference between the biological process of their disease and the repercussions it has on social life and feelings. In a truly holistic way they are part and parcel of the whole problem. However, if the doctor ignores the psychological reactions in favour of the medical pathology, further problems can occur which interfere with treatment and impede recovery.

The common psychological reactions to physical illness vary in type and intensity with no clear point beyond which the reactions will be 'abnormal'. Many of the changes are common and understandable reactions to the social disruption and fears generated by illness.

Whilst severity and type of illness will affect the person's response, the relationship is not clear-cut. Mild problems may give rise to marked emotional changes in one person and in another there will be little or no response to a life-threatening illness. One way of accounting for this variation is to look at the patient's own perception of the problem. This perception will in turn be affected by personality, the nature of the illness and the social context.

The number of different factors may be starting to sound too much to cope with! The point is that the stress of illness has different faces and it is worth looking at these in more detail.

FACTORS INFLUENCING A PERSON'S PERCEPTION OF THE PROBLEM
Personality
Illness is dealt with in different ways according to the person's personality.

The extent to which he or she will experience, remember and complain about pain is affected by whether he or she is naturally highly strung or very outgoing, for example.

The amount of information already received about the situation plays a large part in diminishing uncertainty and anxiety about illness or treatment.

Previous experience of similar problems will supply the sort of information most needed to reduce anxiety. However, if this information comes from seeing apparently similar but actually more serious symptoms in an other person, then very strong but possibly groundless fears may build up.

The person's psychological state at the time of the illness will play a great part in the way he or she perceives its severity. If a gall-bladder problem arises during an anxious time with another member of the family, or the mortgage company start playing up, the experience of the physical illness will be much worse. It is well known that anxiety will lower pain thresholds.

The nature of the illness

There appears to be no direct relationship between the severity of an illness and the possibility of any psychological problem accompanying it. However, the part of the body with the clinical disorder may have a particular significance for the individual. Obvious examples are physical disabilities for sportspersons. It has been suggested that disabling disorders are more threatening for men, whereas disfiguring diseases are more problematical for women. This does not mean to say that this correlation is natural. We are all at the mercy of the roles we take on, the assumptions we have about what makes us attractive or our lives meaningful. What is socially normal may not always be good or sane. Illness, even when extreme, can be an opportunity to grow beyond previously maintained personal boundaries.

The social context

An illness of any severity may have a greater or lesser impact on a person depending on the social context within which it occurs. It may be perceived very unfavourably if it occurs at a bad time, such as starting a new job, whilst it may be accepted as a relief from an unpleasant social situation, such as exams! The reactions of the people around will also play a role in determining the ultimate impact. This can have a direct effect on the perceived severity of a symptom, and may cause a delay before medical help is sought.

THE NATURE OF PSYCHOLOGICAL REACTIONS TO ILLNESS

There are a number of ways in which people respond commonly with major illness. In more sensitive people such responses may happen even after apparently minor problems. The psychological response is one that is unique to the person involved and shouldn't be labelled as hypochondriac. The commonest form this reaction takes are *depression, anxiety* or *denial*.

Depression

This is the commonest response. Studies have shown that between 20 and 30 per cent of all medical patients suffer some degree of depression. This may be relatively mild and seem like a 'flattening' of the emotions together with some loss of interest in the outside world, or it may be pronounced with emotional discomfort, withdrawal and even suicidal feelings.

Depression is often associated with an actual or threatened loss to the person involved. With illness there can be possible losses of parts of the body or losses of bodily and social functions. There are direct parallels between such losses, real or imagined, and the psychological effects of bereavement.

Depression is commonest after the initial stages of an illness when the full implications become apparent. The illness may be interpreted as a punishment for something they have or have not done in the past. Here the depression is commonly coloured by feelings of guilt and self-criticism, especially if the 'punishment' is felt to be justified.

A 'giving-up, given-up complex' commonly happens when the person feels there is little to live for. The feelings are those of hopelessness and helplessness. By helplessness, I mean feelings of impotence and failure or frustration in getting help from the world and people around. Hopelessness refers to the feeling of no longer being able to cope with their problems. Such feelings are common in a short-lived form and pass away when the situation improves. However, for some people these feelings can persist and radically affect both their response to the current illness and openness to subsequent illnesses.

Anxiety

The anxiety commonly associated with illness stems partially from the reasonable uncertainty the patient may have about the cause and outcome of the illness. This will be compounded by inadequate information given by doctors as to the nature of the problem and the treatment prescribed. A herbalist or other practitioner of holistic medicine should not fall into this trap. The anxiety thus produced may be non-specific or may take the form of unnecessary worrying about cause and severity of the illness. As one doctor has put it, 'For the patient, no news is not good news; it is an invitation to fear.'

It usually shows as fear, apprehension and bodily symptoms. They are most prominent in the early stages of the illness and represent a reasonable reaction to the onset of illness and the related uncertainties. It is best to talk freely of your fears and then your medical practitioner should supply clear information. This will not only minimize anxiety but also bring about a better healing response. It is wonderful what trust can do.

Denial

Denial is one way in which people deal with threatening situations and may even be a necessary and adaptive response to the full physical and psychological impact of an illness. It has a protective function by preventing the patient being overwhelmed by anxiety. However, it can go too far when it prevents the person from making a realistic assessment of the severity of his or her symptoms. Thus, denial can be the cause of delay in seeking medical help and so may reduce the chances of a favourable outcome.

Dis-ease and Stress

From all of this it should be apparent that illness does not occur in isolation but happens to an individual with a particular personality and in a particular social context. Both individual and social factors play a role in determining the impact of an illness and the nature of the patient's psychological response can provide considerable insight into his or her underlying personality.

In this chapter we shall consider some of those physical diseases in which psychological factors play an indisputable part. From a holistic perspective such factors are present in all conditions and this approach to health will encompass such mental, emotional and spiritual factors. It is, however, worth looking at the conditions recognized as working in this way so that herbal, dietary and stress management techniques can be seen at work.

In conditions such as heart disease, far more psychological research has been done than in other problems, such as psoriasis. In the discussion that follows there is more information in some sections than others. This does not mean that some problems have more of a stress involvement than others, but simply that more information is available. Herbal guidance is given for the specific diseases, but always in the context of the broader approach to stress and anxiety given elsewhere in the book.

Allergies

An allergy is an abnormally sensitive reaction to a substance in the environment which may not of itself be harmful, but in sensitive people it will trigger the reaction. These so-called allergens can be almost anything, but the commonest are flower or tree pollen, some foodstuffs, household pets and even house dust.

There is a growing recognition that a whole range of conditions appear to be related to 'sub-clinical' allergies, especially to food additives. This is discussed under the section on hyperactivity.

The classic reaction that occurs can take different forms but commonly

appears as hay fever, itching and a rash, a constantly runny nose, wheezing and joint pains. The symptoms are similar with diferent allergies because the body reacts in the same way with the release of a chemical called histamine into the bloodstream.

Times of stress or feelings of anxiety and tension will usually increase the severity or frequency of attacks. With some people, emotional upsets may even be the main factor involved.

Of course the basis of any truly helpful treatment or management of allergic reactions is to stop the exposure to the 'thing' that is triggering it. This can be quite easy where the trigger has been identified as a certain food or animal, but often a simple avoidance is impossible. The commonest treatment is then to use drugs called anti-histamines which suppress the reaction in the body that the allergen is eliciting. For a holistic practitioner of any therapy this is a limited and possibly harmful approach. Acupuncture, homoeopathy and even chiropractic have much to offer in this complaint.

The plant kingdom has been generous in herbs that aid the body in coping with allergies. There are three approaches to the way a herbalist will combat any allergy:

1 Use remedies that help the person get well as a whole person. So not only are anti-allergy remedies used but also those that help any other specific problems unique to that person, all in the context of ensuring health is at a peak. The liver, lungs, kidneys and skin are especially important.

2 These herbs are used in conjunction with an individually worked-out diet (as each person's triggers are unique

to them). Thus, not only will it be based on sound ideas of good nutrition, but will take into account what must be avoided and compensate for any nutritional loss incurred.

3 All the ideas explored in this book to help deal with the impact of stress on that person's life need to be applied in practice. To do this will often involve selecting the most relevant techniques and then setting up a routine for doing them.

There are a multitude of plants that can help in allergic reactions, partially because of the individual nature of the reactions and symptoms. Herbs that ease the symptoms of hay fever – such as itching eyes, runny nose, tight chest – include the following herbs. These should be studied in a complete herbal, as this book concentrates on stress-related plants.

Elder Flower and Berry
All aspects of the elder tree seems to have profound medicinal value. This is why in rural Wales an elder tree was always planted by a new house. If only this was done in modern housing estates! The leaves and the berries are good for sinus catarrh and the itching of the eyes in hay fever. The wine works as well!

Eyebright
As the name suggests, this small meadow flower is renowned as an eye remedy. As a wash it eases discomfort in the eyes.

Garlic
Generally healthy but specific in reducing the impact of allergic reactions.

Golden Rod
One of the best British remedies for sinus catarrh, not only that of allergic origin.

Golden-seal
A specific tonic for the tissue that lines the nose, throat and sinuses. It is generally valuable in allergies that affect these places.

Nettles
Apart from being a painful 'weed', it is a wonderful herb and can reduce allergic tendencies if used regularly.

Peppermint
Will often alleviate the general discomfort of the allergy.

A medical herbalist would also call into play herbs that have an action on a deeper level. These can be quite strong and are best used under professional advice. They include:

Ma Huang
A Chinese remedy that is widely used in Western herbalism as well as Western medicine. Works to reduce the chemical reaction in the blood that is the basis of most allergic reactions. Almost a specific in hay fever and asthma.

Asthma
In an attack, the tubes through which the air is carried in and out of the lungs becomes narrowed. This is caused either by contraction of the muscles in the wall of the tube or also by secretion of a sticky mucus in the tubes themselves. This has the effect of making it more and more difficult to get air in and out of the lungs. This will produce a shortness of breath, wheezing and a cough. The worse the breathlessness, the greater is the feeling of anxiety and even panic. Of course, this will tend to make the attack worse.

CAUSE

The basic physiological problem is a reversible obstruction of the small airways of the lungs. Knowing this, however, does not tell us the precise sequence of the physiological process. An all-encompassing cause for asthma has not been found, but a whole range of triggers are known. Attacks can be triggered in different people by allergies, chest infections, irritant gases, smoke, and psychological factors such as stress and anxiety.

Food allergies are a common predisposing factor. They do not always take the form of overt allergies, and can cause confusion, since taking the food may not trigger an attack – they predispose. The worst culprits here are dairy products; that is, cow's milk, butter and cheese. They are especially implicated in asthma in children who were either not breast-fed or weaned onto cow's milk in the first nine months of life. Other widely involved foods include white sugar, sweets and artificial additives of any kind. It is possible for any food to be involved in individual cases, and specialist help should be sought. There is much that herbal medicine has to offer in the alleviation of allergies but it is best to work with a medical herbalist, whose training includes nutrition and 'clinical ecology', as it is now called.

If a chest infection gets out of hand or occurs in a very prone person, the congestion that develops will trigger attacks. The usual course is for people to get antibiotics from their doctor. However, there are problems with this, especially with young children who may be on repeated courses. A good medical herbalist can help greatly by not only clearing the infection, but by strengthening the lungs and increasing bodily resistance.

Any irritating gas or dust may trigger an attack. This could be smoke from a coal fire or even cold air. By far the commonest and worst such irritant is tobacco smoke. Unfortunately, this is not just from smoking cigarettes but from being around smokers. Anyone with asthma should not feel reticent about asking smokers to abstain in their presence.

PSYCHOLOGICAL FACTORS

Anxiety and stress do not cause asthma, but in most sufferers it can act as an initiating trigger or at least prolong an attack. Usually it will be a combination of factors that produces the attack.

It has been suggested that someone with asthma may often be in conflict with some other key person, commonly a parent, and yet is unable to express any aggressive or hostile feelings in words or actions.

This sort of excessive self-control means that emotional tension is not adequately discharged or cleared, and the asthmatic attack acts as a release of tension along an unusual pathway. This process has been described as 'suppressed crying'. Asthmatics can breathe in but then, in an attack, become unable to breathe *out*, and they seem to choke. Now new air can't be taken in normally. They can't 'let it out'.

The process of 'generalization' can lead to asthmatic attacks in response to a wide range of situations other than the original precipitating one. The understandable anxiety associated with an attack of asthma may itself subsequently lead to a learned automatic response of airway obstruction in a wide variety of anxiety-provoking situations.

TREATMENT

in addition to dietary advice and herbs, interpretative psychotherapy may be useful in helping to deal with emotional problems. Biofeedback techniques have been particularly helpful here in keeping the conscious mind in touch with the body process and so giving a degree of control to the patient. Breathing exercises can be especially helpful in young people. Relaxation and stress management are vital and are discussed in other parts of the book.

A whole range of remedies to help the chest and ease asthma can be used, but it is beyond the range of this book to deal properly with remedies for the lungs. Please refer to a good modern herbal. However, a few can be mentioned.

Grindelia *(Grindelia camporum)*
An excellent herb for easing asthmatic spasm and as a general preventative. It doesn't taste too good!

Wild Cherry Bark *(Prunus serotina)*
This pleasant remedy will reduce spasms and cough and act as a mild relaxant.

Elecampane *(Inula helenium)*
An excellent lung herb that helps clear congestion and strengthen the chest if debilitated.

Herbs that ease nervous tension can be used freely as well as muscle relaxants. Amongst the many described throughout the book it is worth considering:

Cramp-bark *(Viburnum opulus)*
Acts to ease the smooth muscles of the chest and will reduce some of the tension leading to coughing and wheezing.

Motherwort *(Leonurus cardiaca)*
Especially useful because it aids and strengthens the heart as well as easing anxiety.

Scullcap *(Scutellaria laterifolia)*
A generally safe and effective relaxing remedy.

Valerian *(Valeriana officinalis)*
A stronger relaxing remedy that can still be used with safety.

Wild lettuce *(Lactuca virosa)*
A relaxing nervine that will specificaly ease tension in the chest and throat.

Auto-Immune Disease

Many of the more intransigent and baffling of the medical scourges of today are being found to be *auto-immune* in nature. These conditions occur when the body attacks itself with its own defence system. This immune system is very effective and strong, so when misplaced it can cause much havoc.

The name and nature of the disease will vary, depending upon which part of the body is under attack. However, the basis of the problem will be similar in each case and mediated by the immune system. This system is still only slightly understood so I shall make no attempt to explain it. The conditions that may fit in this category range from *rheumatoid arthritis, multiple sclerosis, ulcerative colitis* to *psoriasis*. There is some suggestion that *cancer* may have an auto-immune basis.

Holistic medicine has much to offer in these chronic problems, in that it will help the body as a whole to be as well and integrated as possible. This will often be done by removing from the diet and environment things which act as stressors on the system. These things may be specific foods or inappropriate relationships.

From the evidence that research is rapidly building up, there can be no doubt that mental and emotional stress has much to answer for in auto-immune conditions. Whether it is as a cause or an aggravating factor is not really important. It is, however, vital that ease be brought into the person's life. This may be through relaxation or, perhaps more importantly, the finding of a purpose and meaning in that person's life. Remember the old saying, 'Without vision, the people die.' Maybe this is the key to an understanding of the scourge of auto-immune disease.

Treatment necessitates skilled help.

Blood Pressure

Blood pressure is the pressure created by the heart pumping the blood around the body. As the heart contracts in its beat, the blood pressure in the arteries increases quite abruptly; as the heart relaxes again, the blood pressure drops to about two-thirds of its peak value.

There are always two figures for blood pressure because it is measured at its highest (the systolic) and lowest (the diastolic) points. Peaks of high blood pressure are usually reached several times during the day, but are transient in most people. However, in people with raised blood pressure, these abnormal levels are maintained. There are health risks involved if either the systolic or diastolic pressure are constantly raised.

Periods of stress in people's lives are often associated with a rise in blood pressure. With most people the blood pressure will return to normal if the stress is removed, but with some people this is not the case. If the blood pressure rise has been severe and prolonged, changes can take place in the arteries which result in raised blood pressure being maintained even after the stress has been reduced or removed.

High blood pressure is associated with many other effects. When the pressure is up the heart must pump harder and so is under more strain. This may lead to the oxygen supply to the heart becoming insufficient, which will result in an angina attack. Hardening and narrowing of the arteries becomes much more likely. This may in turn produce heart attacks and strokes as the high pressure can burst blood vessels, resulting in a brain haemorrhage. In extreme cases this may lead to the kidneys becoming affected to the point of kidney failure. From all of this it is clear why high blood pressure is a major health risk, liable to shorten life expectancy considerably.

Blood pressure may become high without any symptoms at all. It is often discovered during routine medical check-ups. It may be heralded by headaches, dizziness, palpitations or unexplained fatigue. If in doubt it is always wise to consult a qualified practitioner, whether 'orthodox' or 'alternative' (an unfortunate and increasingly artificial divide).

The development of high blood pressure probably depends upon a variety of bodily, psychological and environmental factors, all of which are closely interrelated. Even if raised blood pressure is not entirely due to stress, it will be playing an important part. If stress is not a contributing factor at all, which is unlikely, reducing its impact upon life will do nothing but good.

Medical consultation, diagnosis and drug tratment can all play a role in the development of high blood pressure. The side-effects of drugs designed to reduce blood pressure include depression and other psychological disturbances. This, combined with the possibility that knowledge of the diagnosis may itself provoke anxiety, explains the reticence amongst doctors to convey details of blood pressure to patients. From the holistic perspective it is essential that the person with high blood pressure not only be informed of the findings but be intimately involved in the treatment.

This is a vital key in holistic medicine, the acknowledgement that the 'patient' is the truly responsible person involved and the basis of any fundamental healing will come from changes within them. These changes cannot be brought about by drugs or herbs, although both will reduce blood pressure, but through an honest reappraisal of the quality and goals of one's life.

TREATMENT
To treat raised blood pressure effectively there needs to be a reappraisal of life style, diet, degree of relaxation and medicines used.

LIFE STYLE
It is important in the reduction of high blood pressure for the person to learn how to recognize and control stress in his or her life. Approaches to this are discussed in the section on stress. A revaluation of life style and life goals may be called for, and this is often far more effective than any medical treatment, whether herbal, homoeopathic or chemical. Relaxation exercises and possibly meditation have a lot to offer, if the right one is found. Psychotherapy and counselling can be of great value in those people willing and able to benefit from insight into their lives. The techniques that might be used are discussed in depth elsewhere in the book.

DIET
There is commonly a dietary connection in the elevation of blood pressure. The broad approach described for heart problems should be the basis for a diet to combat or prevent high blood pressure. There are some quite specific additional suggestions. Salt should be avoided completely in the food of anyone with blood pressure problems. It should not be used in cooking or added to food on the table. Milk, butter and cheese may contribute to the problem and it is worth cutting them out of the diet completely for at least one month to see if there is a change in the condition. This change will not only show in the blood pressure reading, but as an improvement in the general state of well-being. Oily foods and fats should be avoided.

HERBS
As high blood pressure can be caused by a whole range of factors – from stress and anxiety to kidney failure – there are many herbs that can be used with benefit. There are a number of remedies that have a quite specific role in the normalizing of blood pressure, and two which always come to mind are:

Hawthorn Berries (*Crataegus oxyacanthoides*)
This wonderful remedy acts to tone up the vessels of the whole circulatory system. It has an action that normalizes blood pressure, never reducing it below normal.

Lime Blossom (*Tilia europaea*)
The flowers of this beautiful tree work as a gently relaxant for all stress-related problems, but especially those affecting the heart and blood vessels.

There may be associated water retention

or the suspicion of such, in which case gentle herbal diuretics have a role to play. Whenever medicines are used to help rid the body of water it is always necessary to ensure that there is a supplement of potassium, otherwise there may be a potentially dangerous depletion of this vital mineral. With herbal remedies we can take care of this by using nature's best natural diuretic, Dandelion Leaf (*Taraxacum officinalis*). This will get rid of excess water build-up, but there will be a net increase in potassium in the body. Nature does indeed look after us! Another diuretic that is particularly useful for the circulatory system is Yarrow (*Achillea millefolia*).

A wealth of herbs to help in relaxing both psychological as well as physical tension are available to us. It is worth emphasizing again that the relaxants described here will not replace the development of a more relaxed, less stressed approach to life. The key is being at ease. This is but a partial list of the possible herbs that could be used.

Cramp-bark (*Viburnum opulus*)
A useful relaxing remedy where muscle and body tension accompany a rise in blood pressure. It makes a good external lotion to relax muscle tension or cramp.

Motherwort (*Leonurus cardiaca*)
Apart from its other uses it will help where nervous tension and palpitations accompany the blood pressure.

Scullcap (*Scutellaria laterifolia*)
A widely applicable relaxing nervine.

Valerian (*Valeriana officinalis*)
A strong relaxing remedy that will calm and ease the tension common in this condition. Will also help with sleeplessness.

Wood Betony (*Stachys betonica*)
Especially helpful where there is accompanying headache caused by the rise in blood pressure.

The Digestive System
The whole process of eating and assimilating food is notoriously prone to stress-related problems. Herbal medicine is especially relevant and powerful in the digestive system. A whole range of problems can show themselves, but many have causes in common. Some of the specific diseases will be reviewed here.

PEPTIC ULCER
A peptic ulcer is a breach or defect in the lining of the upper part of the gut. They can occur in the first part of the small intestine (duodenal ulcers), in the stomach (gastric ulcers) or in the gullet (oesophageal ulcers). By far the commonest symptom of all these ulcers is pain followed by heartburn.

Many people with a gastric ulcer find that food will aggravate their pain, whilst those with a duodenal ulcer often find their pain is relieved by eating and brought on by hunger. In both cases the pain is almost always eased by milk or antacids. However, it is not unusual for someone to have 'typical' symptoms without there being an ulcer present.

The origin of peptic ulcers is surprisingly complex and somewhat puzzling, and appears to be different for each type of ulcer, although the strong acid in the stomach plays a leading role. The stomach normally produces a strong acid to aid digestion but protects itself by secreting a coating of mucus.

Food neutralizes stomach acid and it is during periods of stressful work on an empty stomach that the acid begins to damage the lining of the stomach. This will start ulcer formation. Alcohol, and particularly spirits drunk on an empty stomach, will further damage the stomach lining. Smoking affects the stomach in at least two ways: by increasing acid formation, interfering with the secretion of mucus and tiny amounts of swallowed tar and nicotine which directly irritate the lining. Smoking will thus contribute to ulcer formation and slow down its healing.

A number of drugs will aggravate or even cause stomach ulceration. The commonest problem relates to aspirin and the anti-inflammatory drugs used in arthritis. As a general guideline, anyone suffering from indigestion or other stomach problems should avoid anything which contains aspirin or any drug which contains the word 'salicyl–' in the name of its components. It's worth pointing out that originally this group of chemicals was extracted from the bark of willow. The Latin genus name is *Salix* and hence the chemical's name salicylic acid. Willow bark, however, does not cause the problems just mentioned.

Psychological factors may influence the workings of the stomach, either directly through the vagus nerve (the stomach nerve) or by hormones and other biochemical factors. The effects of mood on gastric acid secretion are clear. People with duodenal ulcers tend to respond to the sight and smell of food with greater acid secretion than do others. There is no doubt that stress, anxiety and depression are all pivotal in these digestive conditions.

Treatment

Whilst psychological factors may not be paramount in the causation of ulceration, there can be no doubt that due care and attention to them will speed up remission and reduce any likelihood of relapse. The value of bed rest is not only that it leads to a reduction of gastric acid secretion, but also to the way in which it allows the person to get away from a stressful environment. Successful management must take into account stress, anxiety and depression as well as purely physical factors. Insight psychotherapy may have a lot to offer in helping the individual review and re-evaluate his or her life style and life purpose. At the very least, the use of relaxation techniques to bring ease into that person's life will soften the impact of the problem greatly.

Diet

The basis of dietary advice for peptic ulcers is the need to avoid anything that will act as an irritant. These may be chemical or physical.

Chemical irritants will include acid foods such as vinegar and pickles, any form of alcohol, cigarette smoking, fried and roast food, fizzy drinks, any rich sauces and sweet things. All of these will increase the impact of the stomach acid on the lining and so aggravate the ulcer.

Physical irritants will include too much roughage and extremes of temperature. Even though the virtues of a high-fibre diet are unquestionable, if there is a peptic ulcer present it might act as sandpaper. Where an active ulcer is present it is best to be on a low- or medium-fibre diet. Forget about the F plan! Any drink or food that is too hot or too cold will also irritate and cause pain.

Herbs

Herbal remedies have a lot to offer in all aspects of healing stomach and digestive ailments. The basis of treatment is initially calming down irritation and then promoting the healing of any damaged tissue. A wealth of such herbs is available, each of which acts in a slightly different way. The following are examples:

Comfrey root *(Symphytum officinale)*
A soothing remedy rich in mucilage, but also containing the chemical allantoin which stimulates the healing of wounds. This is the basis of its reputation as the paramount wound herb.

Marshmallow root *(Althae officinalis)*
Another soothing remedy, rich in mucilage, which coats the ulcer and calms down any inflammation present.

Meadow-sweet *(Filipendula ulmaria)*
A natural antacid that acts to reduce the impact of excess acid formation in the stomach.

Slippery Elm *(Ulmus fulva)*
One of the best soothing remedies that is still freely available in chemists' shops.

Other remedies that may prove useful are Sweet Flag, Liquorice root, Irish Moss and Iceland Moss.

As already pointed out, anxiety and tension have a direct impact on the stomach and digestion in general. The nervine herbs have a lot to offer, especially those from the peppermint family (the Labiates) that also contain aromatic oils to settle the digestive system.

Chamomile *(Matricaria chamomilla)*
A gentle relaxing nervine that will ease tension and at the same time act as an anti-inflammatory herb. A remedy that is applicable for all nervous problems of digestion.

Lemon Balm *(Melissa officinalis)*
A wonderfully gentle relaxing herb that is quite safe to use regularly. It will also relieve wind and some sorts of indigestion.

Valerian *(Valeriana officinalis)*
A stronger relaxing nervine that, because of its strong aromatic (though unpleasant) oil, also helps settle wind and indigestion.

Other relaxing herbs that can help are Scullcap, St John's Wort, Pasqueflower, Hops and Passion-flower.

IRRITABLE BOWEL SYNDROME

This is a very common complaint that is also called spastic colon or nervous bowel. It is characterized by colicky pain, which usually occurs in the lower abdomen, a tendency to alternate between diarrhoea and constipation, distension of the abdomen, wind and sometimes heartburn. It may come and go over a very long period of time and is often aggravated by stress and tension.

There are conflicting theories about the causes of this problem, but it appears to be primarily caused by a lack of fibre, roughage, in the diet. This means that by the time the remnants of food reach the colon (large intestine), after the gut has absorbed the nutrients, there is insufficient bulk to enable it to be moved towards the back passage. Instead of small muscular contractions required to squeeze a large bulk down the colon, it has to squeeze very tightly to propel a small bulk. This leads to muscular spasms and so causes pain. The lack of bulk produces either diarrhoea or small, hard stools.

With the muscular spasms going on, any stress causing tension and anxiety will amplify the spasms and aggravate the pain. In fact, stress may just be the extra factor needed to cross the pain and discomfort threshold in the first place.

Treatment

From what has been said it is clear that herbs to help stress and reduce muscular spasms, in addition to a change in diet and a more relaxed approach to life, are the basis of treatment. Relaxation, yoga and meditation have a lot to offer here. A re-evaluation of the person's relationships, work and life purpose will often provide insights that, if acted upon, will remove the health problem.

Diet

Sometimes the simple addition of more roughage to the diet will alleviate the problem, but it is possible to aggravate it if too much bran, or its equivalent, are used too quickly. The increase in fibre is best achieved through eating plenty of green vegetables, salads, fruit and wholemeal bread. It may be appropriate to add bran to breakfast cereal or eat it as bran biscuits. Whilst being a dry, tasteless and boring food it can be made palatable by mixing it with other food. Three tablespoons daily is enough.

Herbs

Nature provides us with remedies that relax the gut as well as soothing the digestive process, in addition to the herbal relaxing nervines for the nervous system itself.

Chamomile *(Matricaria chamomilla)*
A relaxing remedy that will gently ease the tensions in the gut that are causing the gripping pain.

Fennel *(Foeniculum vulgare)*
A carminative that settles gripping, colic and wind through the action of the oils present.

Hops *(Humulus lupulus)*
A moderately strong relaxing herb that is a sedative as well as having a direct anti-spasmodic action on the gut wall.

Peppermint *(Mentha piperata)*
Apart from its wealth of uses, the oil of peppermint is almost specific for calming digestive upsets such as irritable bowel syndrome.

Wild yam *(Dioscorea villosa)*
A remedy that eases spasm and inflammation in the whole of the gut.

The more specifically relaxing remedies should also be considered. These include Valerian, Scullcap and many discussed elsewhere in the book.

COLITIS

A number of difficult problems of the colon are intimately effected by tension and anxiety. These include ulcerative colitis and a less common problem called Crohn's disease. The symptoms are attacks of diarrhoea which contains blood and mucus, associated with pain. Attacks are often precipitated or made worse by stress.

Psychological mechanisms

A lot of research has gone into how psychological factors contribute to ulcerative colitis and it might be worth examining them. It is necessary to distinguish between psychological factors that bring about the onset of an attack, and those which accompany the illness as secondary complications. There appears to be not only a specific type of psychological stress that worsens the condition, but also a pattern of psychological characteristics that act as precursors.

Researchers have claimed that a high

proportion of sufferers have personalities that tend towards being obsessed with someone or something, are easily hurt and find it difficult to express anger. Whilst being outwardly energetic, ambitious and efficient, they inwardly feel insecure and inferior. There also appears to be an excessive dependency on a key person, with whom the relationship is often ambivalent. They have found that not infrequently this person is the mother, who tends to control and dominate. The families of sufferers as a whole tend to be restricted in their interactions and to show a false solidarity.

There appear to be certain sorts of life events more likely than others to trigger off an attack. These are:

1   A real, threatened or fantasized interruption of a key relationship. This could be the loss of someone close, or even the imagined loss. A husband going to work in Saudi Arabia, or the fear of such a move, even though temporary.
2   The expectation of personal performance which the individual feels unable to fulfil. This can take many forms, such as examinations, career goals or relationships.
3   Disapproval from a parent figure – not only real parents, but anyone put into a position of respected authority.

Particularly important as triggers are situations where the person feels hostility and rage whilst also feeling helpless to do anything about it.

This gives a clear example of the way in which specific psychological patterns can contribute to the specific bodily problems. Insight into these non-physical components means that, in addition to physical therapy, the use of counselling will speed up recovery and open up the possibility of avoiding recurrence. It is especially helpful where the person feels unable to cope with his or her life the way it is.

The aim of psychotherapy here should be to help the person become less vulnerable to the stresses of life. In addition there should be an attempt to help that individual develop new ways to deal with the person in his or her life who may be playing the parent-figure role. The themes of dependence and helplessness are ripe for such attention, and whilst sounding impossible to do, psychotherapy can do much to enable change and psychological healing to come about. Another area is in the way that symptoms may be used as a substitute for more efficient ways of dealing with relationship problems. Illness is a good way to gain sympathy and also power over people close by, especially where the illness is all too real.

Treatment
Treatment in these colitis conditions should not be undertaken by unskilled people. Herbal remedies have much to offer in the easing of gut problems. If these are used in the context of working with any anxiety and other psychological patterns, then there is much hope in this distressing and intransigent problem.

Headaches
Headaches must be the commonest complaint to affect us today. Turn on the television at any time and you'll see the most common type of head pain illustrated in advertisements for aspirin or its substitutes. Unfortunately, these drugs offer no lasting relief for chronic pain. If

the roots of the headache are sought and dealt with, the headache will go and not return.

Broadly speaking there are two types of headache, both of which will be aggravated or triggered by stress. There is the muscular tension sort and the vascular or migraine type.

TENSION HEADACHES

Ternsion headaches are not only due to emotional or mental tension. Tight muscles can result from poor posture, from working in awkward positions, and from a too sudden strain. Stress, however, is the commonest catalyst for transforming painless muscle tension into a headache.

As we have seen, the stress can be emotional or perhaps environmental. It could be irritation with the boss or a pneumatic drill outside the window. Whatever the stimulus, the reaction will be the same. The muscles tense to prepare for flight or fight, to get away from the 'threat'. Since we usually don't take any action, the tension builds up until the muscles become sore and cause pain.

Even though we are all under the stresses of our competitive society, not everyone suffers from chronic headaches. Why do some people collapse under the same pressures that others seem to thrive on? Each person has a different stress threshold, which allows one person to cope easily with major life events, whilst another will suffer fits of anxiety in the face of a minor crisis. The anxious person is more prone to headaches.

From this it should be clear that there are a number of better ways to approach headaches than simply taking an aspirin. There are a range of herbal remedies that we shall discuss later, but just as important are attempts to ease the tension that is the root of the pain. This tension may be physical or psychological. A whole range of relaxation exercises are suggested throughout the book. Find one that suits you and use it regularly.

If the problem is more physically based in muscle tension, work with your body. It is possible that your posture, or the position you work in, is the culprit. A common cause of headaches in office workers is cupping the telephone between the shoulder and chin whilst writing. If you are on the telephone a lot, the muscles in your shoulder, neck and head are going to contract and go into spasm. Soon they'll become painful and produce a headache even though you may be feeling calm and relaxed.

There is a simple exercise to help keep the neck and shoulders relaxed and poised. Whenever you feel tension around your head, sit back for a moment and do a few slow head rolls. Bring your chin down to your chest, slowly circle your head to the left, drop it back, bring it to the right and back to your chest. It is best to do five in one direction and then five in the other. These head rolls stretch the muscles that tend to get tense under pressure, this will help relieve any muscle spasms and so any consequent pain.

Herbs for tension headaches

The herbal advice given for the easing of tension will be generally useful for headaches. However, some herbs can produce headaches in sensitive people. The relaxing herb Valerian has been known to do this in some people. Ginseng, *Panax*, may cause headaches if used over too long a period, or at too high a dose.

As such headaches can be caused by a

whole range of factors, there is a similarly wide range of remedies that have reputations in the easing of head pain. It is best to study the associated virtues of the plants and choose those most appropriate in a broader picture. A partial list would include:

Balm	Peppermint
Cayenne	Rosemary
Chamomile	Rue
Elder Flower	Scullcap
Jamaican Dogwood	Thyme
Lady's-slipper	Valerian
Lavender	Wood betony
Majoram	Wormwood

MIGRAINE

Most of the headaches that people describe as migraines are simply severe head pain. These can be bad enough, but migraine describes a specific type of headache due to the contraction and dilation of blood vessels in the membranes that cover the brain. It seems that first a blood vessel constricts, but then the blood flow forces it open again. This dilation irritates the walls of the vessel, causing them to become inflamed and painful. When the blood passes through it produces the characteristic throbbing pain.

A migraine attack may start with visual phenomena which can look like flares around objects, or flashes of zig-zag patterns. The flare, or aura, appears to occur when a blood vessel constricts and causes a loss of blood to the brain. The pain is severe and is often accompanied with nausea and vomiting, as well as a great sensitivity to light.

There appear to be a number of different causes for this traumatic problem. The roots of the migraine may, for example, lie in a spinal problem that could possibly be corrected by an osteopath or chiropractor. The most frequent triggers appear to be food, stress and a change in hormone levels.

For people whose migraine is triggered by stress, the various approaches to stress reduction suggested elsewhere in the book should be tried. Relaxation, meditation and gently soothing exercise can do much to relieve such people. It is well worth taking a close look at environmental conditions such as working under fluorescent lighting or watching a computer VDU all day. The physical environment and the quality of emotional relationships all play a great role in the generating of excess stress.

If there is any suspicion of back, neck, or cranial problems, then it is worth consulting a good osteopath or chiropractor to have these structural factors sorted out. This can often clear the migraines.

It is well established that foods containing tyramine, nitrite, monosodium glutamate or alcohol all have the property of triggering migraines in sensitive people. Many books have been written about the dietary approach to the alleviation of migraine, so here I shall just give the outline of things to avoid. The commonest triggers are:

Cheese
Chocolate
Eggs
Wheat and wheat products
Peanuts
Citrus fruits and tomatoes
Pork.

To avoid these triggers will involve selecting foods that do not contain any of them. In addition to these specific foods, it is worth avoiding tyramine-rich foods. These are:

1 Dairy products: especially cheese, yogurt and sour cream
2 Meat and fish: especially pickled herring, salted fish, sausages, liver.
3 Some vegetables: broad beans, sauerkraut.
4 Alcohol: especially beer, red wine, champagne and sherry.

The last main cause is hormonal changes in women. Migraines that come on at the time of a period or start during menopause, may seem intractable, but can be alleviated by using the right herbal remedies. This should be done by a qualified medical herbalist, however, and is discussed elsewhere.

Herbs
There are many herbs that are reputedly good for migraines. As has been pointed out, to find the right one(s) depends on being sure of the cause. Most of the remedies mentioned for headaches are of value with, perhaps Lavender being a good all-round help. Oil of lavender may be rubbed into the temples, or a couple of drops on a sugar cube could be taken. The flowers can be infused to make a tea. One of Britain's best respected herbalists, Mrs Gosling, FNIMH, has suggested the following easy-to-use mixture as a regular medicine:

Motherwort, Vervain, Dandelion Root, Centaury, and Wild Carrot: each of these mixed together in equal parts and 25 g of this mixture simmered for 15 minutes in 0.5 litres of water. A wineglass of this should be drunk 3 times a day.

The invaluable herb feverfew must be mentioned here. Whilst not quite the wonder remedy the media has led us to believe, the regular use of it – either fresh, as a tablet or as tea – will often clear the migraines, given a month or so of treatment. If you have migraine, then plant feverfew in your garden! It is best to use this herb fresh if at all possible.

Heart Disease

The blood which supplies oxygen and food to the heart moves through the coronary arteries which encircle the heart. If these arteries become narrowed, the blood supply is restricted and may become insufficient. The narrowing is usually due to the deposition on the walls of the blood vessels of a fatty substance called atheroma. If the blood supply is inadequate when an extra load is put on it, for example during exercise or in cold weather, the person may have an angina attack. That is a gripping pain across the chest and sometimes into the neck and jaw or down one or both arms. When the exercise is stopped and the extra demand reduced, the pain will pass in a couple of minutes.

Anxiety, fear and stress may bring on such attacks, as there is an increase in adrenaline and noradrenaline release at such times. These hormones increase the work of the heart, making it beat faster. The pain experienced is itself a stress so that the person will become afraid of having an attack, the heightened anxiety making one more likely.

A heart attack occurs when the blood supply to the heart muscle is abruptly stopped. It is often due to clotting in a coronary blood vessel. As we shall see, stress can contribute to this. The details are not entirely clear, but stress factors increase the stickiness of blood and make it more likely to clot.

The origins of these common problems are complex and confusing. Some of the factors involved are well known and can lead to clear guidelines for possible prevention, but simplistic statements about saturated fats or jogging can be misleading. The search for factors that contribute to the scourge of heart disease has highlighted diet, socio-economic conditions, psychological and behavioural characteristics and life events.

FOOD

Whole forests have been turned into pulp to provide paper for the articles about cholesterol, polyunsaturated fats and heart disease. Anyone trying to read them all, or even follow the broad arguments, will get very stressed from the disagreements!

From the wealth of research done, it has been shown that heart disease has definite links with too much fat in the diet, raised blood cholesterol, raised blood pressure, smoking, obesity, short stature and underactivity. The precise role of these factors is unclear, but general guidelines about a possible preventive diet appear.

Something that is certain is the involvement of fats. Whilst the so-called saturated fats may be the worst, it seems that it is an over-preponderance of all fat in the total diet that is to blame. The way in which stress interacts with fats is partly as follows: A stressful existence leads to the sustained production of the hormones adrenaline and noradrenaline. Among their actions, they mobilize fatty acids from the body's fat store, which provide a rapid source of energy. However, in the absence of exercise to burn up these fatty acids, it is thought that they accumulate and interact with other fatty substances to form a fatty substance called atheroma which is deposited in plaques on the walls of blood vessels. This is most critical in the blood vessels close to the heart and in the brain and kidneys, because it will cause a narrowing of the vessels and so limit the amount of blood available.

In this book we shall not explore specific diets in much depth, but these ideas are basic to heart problems:

1 Animal fats and cholesterol-rich foods should be kept to a minimum. These include red meat, dairy products and eggs.
2 An absolute minimum of salt. Ideally don't add any to food, either in cooking or on the table.
3 DON'T SMOKE!
4 Excessive alcohol should be avoided.
5 Generally avoid becoming overweight.
6 Avoid refined food, white sugar and white bread, and artificial additives of any kind.

PERSONALITY

An association between a particular type of personality and heart disease has been suggested for many years. As early as 1959 researchers were able to show that there was a difference in the risk of developing heart disease between two types of behaviour; these were called type A and type B.

Type A behaviour is characterized by a chronic sense of time-urgency, aggressiveness which may be repressed and striving for achievement. Type A people will often drive themselves on to meet deadlines, many of which will be self-imposed. There are feelings of being under pressure of time and responsibility, often doing two or three things at once. They are likely to react with hostility to anything that seems to get in their way and are temperamentally incapable of letting up. They are liable to think of themselves as indispensable. All of which adds up to a state of constant stress!

Type B behaviour is the opposite of these characteristics. They are less preoccupied with achievement, less rushed and generally more easy-going, not allowing their lives to be governed by a sense of deadlines. They are less prone to anger and do not feel constantly impatient, rushed and under pressure. They are also better at separating work from play and know how to relax.

Studies done over a period of eighteen months to two years with a group of type A and type B people showed that there was a 31 per cent increased risk of developing heart disease in type As.

Many physical differences have been show in people who exhibit these two types of behaviour. For example, there appear to be more deposits in the coronary arteries of people that fit into the type A category than type B. This has a close association with other medical risk factors, such as smoking, shortened blood-clotting time, higher than normal blood fat levels, increased daily secretion of adrenalin which in turn increases the oxygen requirement of the heart muscles and releases fatty acids from the body fat.

There is much debate on the methods for assessing type A behaviour, the details of which do not concern us here. The important insight is the association of types of behaviour with disease development. However, there are *not* two types of people! Each person is an individual, and whilst people can always be fitted into artificial categories, these categories do not identify them.

SOCIO-ECONOMIC FACTORS

A number of social and economic factors can be associated with an increased risk of heart disease; however, the findings tend to vary according to the society being studied. Some studies emphasize high risk in upper socio-economic groups whilst others stress the opposite. Some evidence suggests that class variation disappears when the degree of physical activity is taken into account.

High risk factors appear to be:

1 Social mobility – change of environment such as house move or change of job.
2 Social incongruity – inconsistency in status relevant to the person's life situation.

The relatively low occurrence of heart disease in women appears to be due to psychosocial rather than biological factors. Men with an exaggerated striving for dominance and who use work as a major outlet for aggression are more exposed to particular stresses and conflict and are more conditioned than women to 'control' emotions when dealing with such conflict.

Such patterns seem to explain the difference between the occurrence in Western societies and those of the Third World. The work pressures have hitherto been less intense, with family and social stability supporting the man and not exposing him to the frustrations that characterize the pattern described above.

Many ideas have been put forward to try and explain Western civilization's predisposition to heart disease. For example:

1 It occurs through the imposition of the need for self-discipline governed

by intellectual control and distant goals rather than basic drives and their more immediate gratification.

2 It has been suggested that the modern environment encourages high-risk type A behaviour by rewarding haste, aggressive competition, and a constant excessive preoccupation with the demands of work schedules.

LIFE EVENTS

Particularly stressful times in a person's life will act as possible danger points in any stress-related problem such as heart disease. When these are identified, it is possible to take them into account and plan ahead. This makes it possible to manage and lessen the impact of the stresses on health and well-being. There are well-known points of increased stress in everyone's life and they have been called life events. They are especially important in conditions such as angina and heart disease. They are discussed in depth in another chapter of the book.

TREATMENT

The treatment of heart disease must be undertaken by a skilled practitioner. To do the best that is possible it is essential, however, that the sufferer of the condition be involved in its treatment. This might sound like a truism, but unfortunately we have become isolated from our own healing process by the very expertise of the doctors and even the herbalists.

This is especially so when the emotional and mental aspects are considered and from a holistic perspective it is obvious that the psychological aspects of treatment and recuperation must be taken into account. It comes as no surprise that a great reduction in the chance of any repeat occurrence of the attack or the development of complications follows the management of psychological and social problems.

Ways of dealing with tension and anxiety must be found that will suit the person involved. There are many different ways of relaxing and not all of them suit everyone. The ways in which this can be done are considered elsewhere, but the individual may need help with anxiety and tension which can have its roots in self-image, belief systems, relationships, work goals and environment, etc. Treatment should be based on a broad reappraisal of life style and life goals, not simply in medical approaches to the illness. Diet, exercise, relaxation, meditation, etc. are all potentially appropriate and described throughout the book.

Herbs

Herbal remedies have a lot to offer in the treatment, prevention and alleviation of heart problems. *It must be stressed, however, that any herbal treatment of the heart must be undertaken under the supervision of a well-trained medical herbalist*, especially if the heart is already being treated with drugs.

There are a number of remedies that have a direct action on the heart itself. These include the following:

Broom *(Sarothamnus scoparius)*
Hawthorn berries *(Crataegus sp.)*
Lily of the valley *(Convallaria majalis)*
Lime blossom *(Tilia europaea)*
Mistletoe *(Viscum album)*

You will notice that I haven't included the well-known heart herb Foxglove. In modern medical herbalism this is considered too poisonous and is only used under certain circumstances. It should never be used in the home.

A whole range of herbs can be used to aid and support the heart through generally helping the body by their actions elsewhere.

There is much that can be done with herbs to help the anxiety and tension that accompanies and contributes to heart problems. These are all considered in much more depth in other parts of the book, but it is worth pointing out one that has particular relevance where the heart is involved in stress. It is:

Motherwort (*Leonurus cardiaca*)

Its Latin name shows how its reputation for aiding the heart has been incorporated into botany. It may be used where there are palpitations. Other relaxing plants that may prove useful include the following; remember, however, that different remedies may suit some people more than others:

Balm (*Melissa officinalis*)
St John's wort (*Hypericum perforatum*)
Scullcap (*Scutellaria laterifolia*)

Hyperactivity in Children

This is a growing area of concern, as its causes seem so all-pervasive. It is clear that artificial food additives have a lot to answer for here. It appears that young, developing nervous systems are particularly prone to the damage or irritation that many food additives can cause. The effect is one of excessive activity with only a few hours sleep each night, and because of the over-activity the sufferers are more prone to accidents. There is some association with eczema and asthma, both of which will be aggravated anyway by the overactivity. There may be difficulties with speech, balance and learning, even if the child has a high IQ.

Anyone with a child that is suspected of having this problem will be under extreme stress themselves. So there are two things to look at: ways to help the child and ways for the parents to cope.

An excellent support and help group – Hyperactive Children's Support Group – has been formed that is a mine of useful information in this problem. They can be contacted at the following address (but send an s.a.e): Mrs Sally Bunday, 59 Meadowside, Angmering, West Sussex, BN16 4BW. In USA contact: The Feingold Association, 56 Winston Dr, Smithtown, NY 11787 (516 543-4658).

A treatment that can be quite effective is based on a diet by Dr Feingold and cuts out all foods and drink containing synthetic additives of any kind and certain natural chemicals. For more specific details contact the Support Group above.

However, there are specific food additives to avoid, and these are by law marked on any package containing them. They are:

E102 Tartrazine	154 Brown FK
E104 Quinoline Yellow	155 Brown HT
107 Yellow 2G	E210 Benzoic
E110 Sunset Yellow	acid
E120 Cochineal	E211 Sodium
E122 Carmoisine	benzoate
E123 Aramanth	E250 Sodium
E124 Ponceau 4R	nitrite
E127 Erythrosine	E251 Sodium
128 Red 2G	nitrate
E132 Indigo Carmine	E320 Butylated
133 Brilliant blue	hydroxyanisole
E150 Caramel	E321 Butylated
E151 Black PN	hydroxytoluene

These are additives that there is little doubt about, but the complete list of possible culprits is almost endless.

A combination of the diet and good herbal treatment for any bodily symptoms the child has developed should be able to clear the problem.

Herbal relaxants that may help include the following that may be best used as an infusion added to a bath; the way to do this is described in the section on preparations:

Red Clover
A gentle relaxing remedy that helps aid the liver and also clears the skin of minor eruptions.

Lime Blossom
A stronger though still mild, relaxing herb.

Chamomile
An all-round relaxing plant for children.

Having said that, it is the parents who often need herbs for stress and tension, more than the children. Any parent supporting a hyperactive child would benefit from the advice given in the section on how to deal with long-term stress.

Insomnia
Good sleep is fundamental to good health and lack of sleep will hurt either immediately or eventually. On a day-to-day basis, pain, stress and anxiety may all be disruptive to a good night's sleep, leaving you fatigued the next day. This fatigue will reduce the body's ability to cope with stress and discomfort, so that you are even more uncomfortable and probably more anxious. This makes it more likely that the following night's sleep will be spoiled. And so you enter into a vicious cycle of stress – anxiety – insomnia – fatigue – increased stress and pain.

The lack of enough sleep may be voluntary, staying up late to watch late television or to go to a party, for example. Getting less sleep than you should for extended periods may also be by choice. It may appear that the body has apparently adapted to operating on a tired basis. However, this will tell in the long run via serious disease or disorder, increasing vulnerability to stress symptoms, and faster ageing.

HERBS TO HELP SLEEP
Nature is rich in plant remedies that help sooth the sometimes stormy route to sleep. If the mind won't stop or the body is too agitated, or for no good reason at all, herbs can be of much help.

The strong and potentially dangerous narcotic plants are, of course, illegal and won't be discussed here. All the plants mentioned are safe and non-addictive.

They can be used in a number of ways. The specific details are discussed in the section on preparations, but to aid sleep they are most effective as teas or used as additives in baths. This works best with relaxing plants that have a pleasant aroma. The combination of a relaxing nervine herb such as a few drops of Lavender Oil added to the bath, followed by a cup of sleep-inducing Valerian tea is both pleasant and effective.

All the relaxing remedies discussed later in the book may be sufficient to help relax the body and mind enough for sleep to come. Herbs such as Scullcap, Lavender, Motherwort, whilst primarily not for insomnia, may have the desired effect. Here I shall list the plants with a reputation for inducing sleep.

Hops
A traditional remedy still used in the form of hop pillows to help with sleep. A tea is usually used.

Jamaican Dogwood
A good relaxing remedy that also has mild pain-relieving properties.

Lime Blossom
A gentle relaxing remedy that is safe with children. It makes a good herb pillow in the style of hops. Especially good for its beneficial effects on the circulation.

Passion-flower
One of the best sleep-producing plants that is used in most proprietary mixtures. The right dosage varies, so experiment, building up the strength over a few nights.

Valerian
A good relaxing nervine that can be used during the day for anxiety and tension and at night to aid sleep where this is disturbed by anxious thoughts. However, this herb does not suit everyone, so if you get headaches or do not feel at all better, do not continue with it. Try another.

Wild Lettuce
With some people this remedy can be a strong sedative, but not always, unfortunately.

With the wide range of plants that can help and the different ways to use them, it would need a separate book to explore all the ramifications of herbs for sleep. There are a few favourites that I have.

A mixture of equal parts of Scullcap, Valerian and Passion-flower makes an effective sleep potion. It can be made by mixing equal parts of the dried herb or the tinctures. If using the dried herb, then an ounce of the herb mixture to a pint of boiling water should be left to infuse for ten minutes. If the insomnia is a major problem, then take a wine-glassful of the tea after each meal and two before going to bed.

In addition to herbal remedies some dietary changes can help. For example, a light snack an hour before going to bed may help some people, especially if it's a lettuce sandwich – perhaps because it is the cultivated cousin of the wild species.

The natural amino acid L-Tryptophan taken regularly for about a month will usually help the sleep process. It is a natural precursor to a sleep-inducing chemical found in the brain. Another supplement that can help is taking Dolomite tablets. In addition, remember the guidelines for diet and low stress. Don't take any caffeine drinks such as tea, coffee, hot chocolate or cola from 5 p.m. onwards, as these will tend to keep awake those with a sleep problem.

RELAXATION FOR SLEEP
The relaxation exercises discussed in that section of the book will help you ease into sleep. Give them a try. For some people, the relaxation and sleep-aiding tapes that are now available prove quite useful.

If you use the exercises described in this book to help you fall asleep, continue until you either fall asleep or complete the entire exercise. If you actually complete the routine and yet you are still mentally awake, don't be concerned about not being asleep, because by this time you body is deeply relaxed. You are getting excellent physical rest anyway, and it's usually true that if you're this relaxed and haven't fallen asleep, then your brain apparently doesn't really need the sleep at this time.

In this situation, try and enjoy yourself: dream, fantasize, speculate, ponder decisions that need making, consider problems that need solving, and so forth. You're relaxed, so don't be afraid to entertain any subject of thought. Many people find this physically calm, mentally clear state very attractive and productive. If you think of something you want to write down, get up and do so. You won't spoil any magical physical state. In fact, upon returning to bed you may fall asleep more readily than ever.

Usually you will fall asleep long before completing the slow, complete relaxation. In fact, you may wake up the next morning and not remember getting any further than the legs!

So while you're lying waiting to fall asleep, you'll focus on breathing and muscle awareness and relaxation. Don't be concerned with when and if you actually fall asleep. Remember, you can't control that, anyway. And any attention you give to such thoughts as 'Am I asleep yet?' doesn't help you to fall asleep any sooner, and may help you worry into staying awake longer. Instead of focusing on whether you're asleep yet, or what discomforts you feel, or what house sounds you can hear, focus on breathing and muscle awareness each night until you are either asleep or so deeply relaxed physically that it doesn't matter.

MORE THOUGHTS ON SLEEP

Never try to fall asleep. Sleep isn't done, it just happens when your mind and body are ready. The best you can 'do' is clear the things that may be keeping you awake, such as unconscious muscle tension. If you're both mentally and physically restless and can't get comfortable, don't fight it – get up and do something, anything, for a short while, even though you're not really interested – force yourself. You'll soon feel quite tired.

Do the exercises lying on your back, even though you may be used to falling asleep on your side. Either you'll fall asleep on your back, which is good for you, or you'll turn onto your side as you lose focus and begin to drift off.

Use pillows in such a way that your neck and head extend straight up from your spine, without twisting or bending sharply.

Be sure your bedding is firm enough to support your body evenly, especially along the spine, without sagging.

Do not eat for at least three to four hours before going to bed. Drink may be all right, but definitely no food or caffeine drinks. Eating not only stimulates your metabolism just when it should be slowing down, but it is also a major factor in gaining excess weight. The only exception would be the lettuce sandwich mentioned above.

If you wake up in the middle of the night, and don't fall back to sleep within ten to fifteen minutes, then simply begin the relaxation exercises again.

Pain

It may come as a surprise, but pain is not an illness. It is a subjective sensation, and has been described as an emotion. It is usually an accompaniment to some bodily ill and often acts as an early-warning sign. As such, pain plays a valuable role in health – not that it should be welcomed, but rather listened to. This is the most worrying aspect of the enormous consumption of pain-killers today. Much is being masked and suppressed that should be listened to, not only physical ills but those of emotional pain as well. Much pain can have its roots in the subtleties of body language, with the pain acting as body semaphore for mental and emotional warning signs.

The very relative experience of pain will often be amplified or reduced by previous experience of pain and its relief and the person's ability (or inability) to cope with it. Physical pain may become much worse when the person is worrying and anxious about their illness.

As with all other bodily manifestations, pain will be worse under all forms of stress. A good example would be a backache worsened as a result of anxiety about a bank overdraft.

Different people will have varying degress of pain tolerance and it is profoundly difficult to comprehend another's experience of pain. Pain can cause anxiety and depression, especially when associated with chronic illness.

TREATMENT

From what has been said, it should be clear that pain as such is not what the healer should focus on. Primarily it should be the roots of the pain that are seen to, and pain-killers used only within a broader treatment of the pain's cause.

Appropriate treatment might lie in the hands of a chiropractor or osteopath for any pain related to structural problems. Acupuncture has a lot to offer. It is becoming increasingly clear that many headaches have their origin in jaw problems that good dentists may be able to help with.

Herbal remedies are the basis of most of the pharmaceutical drugs used today. All the morphine and cocaine type pain-killers and anaesthetics come originally from plants. None of the strong anodynes are freely available, for obviously they must only be used under

qualified observation. In the current state of medical monopoly this restricts properly qualified medical herbalists from using such herbs, an unfortunate state of affairs.

There are some gentle herbs that can relieve pain, but to underline the point, the cause of the pain must be sought. Safe herbs worth considering include the following:

St John's Wort

This is especially valuable for long-standing neuralgic pain, used internally or as an external application for at least three weeks.

Jamaican Dogwood

Also a mild sedative.

Valerian

It will aid in anxiety reactions that might accompany the pain.

Yellow Jasmine

This is a much stronger pain reliever that should be used only under skilled herbal advice.

Wild Lettuce

A good relaxing pain reliever, although the wild variety is now rather rare.

The above plants are for pain in general, but that is not very common! If pain is due to muscle spasms then try anti-spasmodic herbs; if due to external problems use vulnerary ones. The complete list would be almost endless here, but bear in mind that anxiety will aggravate and be aggravated by pain.

Rheumatoid Arthritis

This increasingly prevalent disease is undoubtedly aggravated by stress of any kind. As already pointed out, it is one of the so called *auto-immune* conditions, all of which will be worsened by anxiety and tension.

Rheumatoid arthritis is characterized by swelling, pain and stiffness of joints in the body. However, it is quite different in origin to the more common *osteo-arthritis*. In rheumatoid there is a proliferation of inflammatory tissue in the membranes that line some of the body's joints. The specific cause is unknown but is directly related to the body's immune system. It is the immune system that defends the body against disease organisms. For some reason, in rheumatoid arthritis the defence process is started up against the body's own protein in the joint lining. This causes the painful inflammation and eventual destruction of tissue.

TREATMENT
Amongst factors that disturb the immune system in prone people is the impact of stress, so any effective treatment of this difficult illness must include stress management that is relevant to the individual involved. An easing of tension and anxiety must be a priority.

Diet also plays a role in the aggravation and possibly even the origin of rheumatoid arthritis. The possible ramifications of this are complex, so advice should be sought from a skilled practitioner. The basics are low acid and no dairy products with an avoidance of *all* artificial additives. The role of diet in the treatment of rheumatoid arthritis is a complex and contentious area. A list of books is included in the bibliography.

Herbal medicine has a lot to offer, but as this is a deep-seated problem based in the immune system it is impossible to talk of specific remedies. A good herbalist will be of much help. The following plants have a role in any broad treatment, which must take into account the unique situation of the patient involved. Remember that to truly help, the whole person's condition must be treated, and they may suffer from more than just the named joint condition.

Black Cohosh
A useful cleansing and relaxing herb that aids in reducing inflammation.

Bogbean
One of the best all-round remedies for arthritic conditions in the body. It also acts on the liver and aids digestion and general body cleansing.

Celery Seed
An excellent remedy that has a specific affinity for the skeleton and musculature. Celery is worth becoming a major part of the diet of any one prone to arthritis.

Meadow-sweet
A useful all-round remedy that amongst its wealth of attributes works to reduce inflammation in the joints.

Wild Yam
A herb that is the natural origin of synthetic steroids. It can aid in acutely inflamed arthritis. Used in digestive problems such as diverticulitis.

Willow Bark
A rich source of natural aspirin that does not have any of the potential problems of the synthetic drug. Can be used to ease the pain in the joints.

Skin Disease
The skin often acts as a lightning conductor, grounding stress through the body from the mind to express itself on the surface. It is as though it is a form of body semaphore. It often is a cry for help or attention, which the person will

usually deny as such. It is this very denial that makes it necessary for the skin manifestation to appear. In this perception lies a powerful way of approaching skin disease. Through counselling and supportive psychotherapy much can be done to ease the impact of conditions such as psoriasis and so reverse the momentum of the illness and speed its clearing.

The skin is affected by many different things, from simple infections, through allergies to the more complex and obscure auto-immune problems. Most skin conditions will be aggravated by anxiety and tension and some actually brought on by stress itself. This is especially true of a form of eczema called atopic eczema and psoriasis. Whilst psoriasis is not an emotional based illness as many consider it to be, it will of itself act as an emotional stress. In fact, this emotional stress caused by psoriasis is often one of the worst features of the condition.

Emotional factors and stress are important in the development, aggravation and perpetuation of many skin diseases, and the stress and even misery caused by a skin disease may lead to a vicious circle. An awareness by friends, relatives and the general public that such conditions are not contagious, that it is not dirty, that it is not the sufferer's fault and that it causes them great embarrassment, would help to reduce stress caused by skin disease and make the treatment a lot easier.

All holistic approaches to medicine have a lot to offer in treating skin disease. Dietary approaches are especially indicated in skin problems, but this is an area that goes beyond the range of this book. Used internally as systemic acids and externally as ointments and lotions, herbal remedies are particularly helpful. The list of possible remedies is endless, but here are some suggestions:

Burdock Root
A good general remedy for chronic skin problems that will also aid digestion and assimilation of food because of the way it works on the liver. Especially useful in psoriasis and rheumatism.

Chickweed
As a lotion, ointment or in a bath it will reduce irritation, sometimes quite dramatically.

Cleavers
A common plant that specifically works on the lymphatic system and so helps in one of the body's own cleansing systems. Useful in all skin problems.

Figwort
A widely useful herb for skin problems that acts as a general tonic.

Golden-seal
One of our herbs that comes close to being a 'cure all'! Because of its broadly beneficial action on the body it will aid in most skin problems and is a good lotion in eczema and skin infections like ringworm, especially combined in equal parts with marigold or myrrh.

Marigold
The flowers used internally or externally are especially useful in eczema. One of the best wound healers and specific for fungal infections.

Myrrh
This 'old-fashioned' remedy is still available in all chemists' shops and makes a good external wash for infections.

Yellow Dock
Good for chronic skin conditions and also a mild laxative.

This is a small selection of the plant remedies available. In addition there are all the nervine relaxant herbs that are explained elsewhere. One that is worth a special mention here is:

Red Clover

A gentle skin remedy that is specific in some types of childhood eczema. It also has a mild relaxing actions and aids a restful sleep, reducing itching and thereby causing less scratching.

Some Specific Stress Problems of Women

In Western society, all kinds of emotional and mental disorders are commoner in women than men. This bald fact opens up vast areas of psychological, sociological, physiological and political exploration, most of which is inappropriate to discuss now. The main suggested reasons for the difference are genetic and the social pressures on women and differences in patterns of upbringing and cultural expectations. The works of feminist writers such as Germaine Greer in *The Female Eunuch* will show how such difference are produced and maintained. Suffice it to say that something is wrong with a society that causes such suffering in half its population.

Whilst we shall focus on the medical 'syndromes' common to women, it must be remembered that the atmosphere of mental illness that pervades our society can be easily seen as a result of the patriarchy that runs it. The alienation and depersonalization of the high-rise, militarism, multinational corporate oppression, the nuclear threat and inequality of world resources leading to massive misery could all be seen as aspects of male mental disorders. This could get too political, but to view health holistically means that such perspectives cannot be avoided.

Perhaps there should be some attention given to male menopause and the male version of pre-menstrual tension. Whilst that might sound like a joke, I'm afraid there is something to it!

It might be a bit pretentious for a male herbalist to try and comprehend how herbs can help with 'female' problems. What I shall focus on are those health problems that most commonly feed patterns of stress and anxiety and the ways herbs can ease them. The broader issues of relationships and cultural roles I shall but hint at.

A herbal that is full of a deep compassion and comprehension in this area is '*Hygieia*' by Jeannine Parvati. I strongly recommend its insights.

PRE-MENSTRUAL TENSION

This is a condition that until recently was denied official existence! It was put down to 'hysterical female behaviour', of course, by male doctors.

It can be described as a condition of physical, behavioural and mood changes related to the menstrual cycle. The commonest symptoms include irritability, depression, breast tenderness and a 'bloated' sensation. Such changes are found in many cultures and ethnic groups. During the pre-menstrual period there is an increased rate of appeals to suicide prevention centres and women are more likely to enter hospitals as psychiatric emergencies. Pre-existing disorders such as migraine or skin problems are likely to be exacerbated pre-menstrually. Life generally becomes more of a strain, the degree of pressure varying between women.

Little clarity has come from physiological research about the root causes of this problem. Localized water retention in various parts of the body has been implicated as a possible cause of the tension, as have hormonal changes. Cyclical changes in certain brain chemicals have been suggested in the same way. There is no doubt that marked body changes occur at all levels of study.

All such physiological work ignores, to its loss, the powerful involvement of mind and emotion in PMT and menstruation in general. There is a suggestion that pre-menstrual and menstrual problems are a conditioned pattern of response to the hormonal changes resulting from the woman's experience of her mother's attitudes and approaches to periods. If these attitudes were not open and healthy, then as a child the girl would develop resistance and psychological blockage around the whole subject. As she grew and matured this would surface as pre-menstrual tension. There are many other such theories, the point being that this disruptive and unpleasant problem has a range of causative factors feeding it. There is no one thing to blame.

Treatment

Herbal medicine can prove extremely successful in the short-term relief and long-term improvement of PMT.

Scullcap

This valuable remedy can be considered a specific for the relief of the emotional and mental symptoms of PMT. This may be combined with a whole range of the effective tension-relieving remedies that we have available to us. This could include the following:

Cramp-bark

A generally mild relaxing herb but very effective in easing the cramps that may be associated with PMT.

Motherwort

May be useful in combinations because of its relaxing properties plus its safe action of reducing stress-related palpitations.

Pasque-flower

A valuable relaxing plant that will help where there is a degree of tearful emotion that becomes too much. Tears are good for you, though!

Valerian

Widely used with benefit in PMT, especially where there is any cramping pain or over-agitation.

The specific remedies chosen will depend on those that work best, obviously, but also on the degree of associated cramping or water retention, etc. This might all start sounding a bit complex, but in fact is quite straightforward. Such herbs as Scullcap for PMT are best used when the problem is active just before the menstruation starts.

Long-term treatment is best based on the use of Chasteberry in the context of a balanced herbal approach to the person's whole being. It works over a period of time to balance hormone levels without interfering with any of the body's necessary work.

Herbs that remove water from the body, diuretics, are sold in chemist's shops for the relief of PMT. The value of diuretics is debatable, as the water retention may be secondary to the emotional tension rather than the other way around. Thus Scullcap may relieve the water retention whilst diuretics may not ease the tension. If diuretics are suggested, then consider: Dandelion Leaf; Bearberry; Yarrow.

These are only suggestions, each woman is unique and occasionally the 'specifics' do not do a thing.

The use of vitamin B12 has been advocated and is widely suggested by GPs; however, the evidence is equivocal.

Both supportive and insight psychotherapy have a valuable role, as do relaxation and possible medication techniques, all of which are discussed elsewhere in the book.

PSYCHOLOGICAL PROBLEMS OF PREGNANCY

Pregnancy is such a wonderful experience of life in the raw, yet also in the 'soft'! If only men could——!

Having seen the impact that 'life events' can have on emotional and mental problems, during pregnancy there is a reduced chance of a woman developing severe mental problems. Of course, this is as it should be, highlighting the inherent health and wholeness of this most holistic of 'life events'.

Pregnancy, particularly the first one, is a psychological watershed. The transition to motherhood is a creative process in which fundamental changes in the concept of self and of role are negotiated against a background of resolved and still unsettled developmental 'crises'. The psychological and physical demands of the infant are an essential ingredient in this process of maturation which begins, however, long before the baby is born. For the pregnant woman, becoming a mother means becoming a different sort of child of her own parents, a different sort of sexual partner, and, indeed a different sort of mother if there are already other children. Temporary or permanent changes of career and of social role can be a direct consequence of pregnancy and are sometimes a source of major difficulty.

Apart from women with a previous history of mental ill health, the minor problems that do arise can be dealt with by increased support from midwives, doctors and herbalists, but most especially from the family. There is a need for clear and informed reassurance, antenatal classes and sharing with other mothers.

Ten to 35 per cent of pregnant women take some form of tranquillizer or sleeping pill. All of the drugs that can cross the blood-brain barrier will also cross into the placenta. Higher blood levels will develop in the foetus than the mother, and this will lead to sedation of the baby. The inappropriateness and danger of this should be made clear. The use of supportive counselling, marriage therapy and herbal nervines is obviously preferable.

Problems associated with miscarriage, stillbirth, or abortion will greatly benefit from the help of an experienced and skilled counsellor.

All the herbs that will ease anxiety and tension are usually quite safe for use during pregnancy, but if needed often it is best to consult a qualified practitioner.

POST-NATAL DEPRESSION

About 10 per cent of women develop a depression in the time just after childbirth. Onset is usually within the first month. Investigations to find metabolic causes are inconclusive, but it is often easy to point to psychological and social factors such as marital disharmony, poor housing, financial problems. In one research project, it was found that post-natal depression happens more frequently in women who had doubts about continuing with their pregnancies or in those who had described difficulties in relationships with their own parents.

Such depression may have repercussions on the child. Any difficulties in adjusting to being a mother are likely to be exacerbated by the symptoms of depression, e.g. increased irritability, lowered self-esteem, guilt, inability to cope.

Management of post-natal depression
Such depression usually passes within a few months and this will be considerably speeded by simple supportive measures. This would include reduction of any sense or experience of isolation, identification of sources of stress and then their avoidance or removal. Sharing of feeding responsibilities often helps both parents in this time of profound re-orientation. What should be a time of joy and coming together so often becomes one of stress and tension.

However, some mothers express inner conflicts by an inability to allow the child a separate existence. Thus they scrutinize the baby's every movement and although complaining about exhaustion and misery they are resistant to counselling and support.

Apart from such support, advice to ensure adequate diet and appropriate herbal medication will ease matters. The herbs may be other than nervines and anti-depressants, as there is a need to aid the body in its task of recuperation and breast-feeding. Qualified herbal advice must be sought for this.

MENOPAUSE
The menopause is one of the biggest transitions a human being can go through. Much has been written and much said about its multiple problems; however, it can be a time of release and freedom. The ties of a lifetime and roles with which society has bound women can be loosened.

The undoubted physical problems of the hormonal transformation can be eased and in some cases removed altogether. Whether the hormonal changes lead to the rather too common mental and emotional problems is unclear. However, it is a time of major life events – children leaving home, parents dying, husband retiring, etc.

There can be no doubt that this time period has profound implications for the women involved, the major changes in personal role often being seen as her becoming 'useless'. Valuable counselling work can be done based on an exploration of the opportunities that open up in the 'change of life', as a new start where the woman can create what she wants and not simply what her children and husband need, if previously these defined her activities. It can be a release rather than a rejection, no matter what she is changing *from* and moving *to*.

Herbal medicine can help with both the hormonal and the psychological problems. Herbs to consider include:

Blue Cohosh
An American Indian plant that balances and normalizes the function of the whole of the female reproductive system.

Chaste-berry
A valuable remedy from the Eastern Mediterranean that balances hormonal traumas and has a profound action in lessening the 'hot flushes'.

False Unicorn Root
Similar in broad action to Blue Cohosh.

Golden-seal
An excellent remedy for all-round health and specifically for the toning of mucous membranes, such as those that line the womb and vagina.

Lady's-mantle
Named from its leaf shape, it has similar properties to Chaste-berry, although not as strong.

Life Root
Similar in broad action to Blue Cohosh.

A whole range of the herbal relaxing and anti-depressant remedies may be indicated. The specifics will vary from woman to woman and so should ideally be prescribed by a good herbalist. Certain plants are worth emphasizing:

Motherwort
A nervine that can be most useful where the flushes are compounded by palpita-tions. A safe, relaxing remedy.

Pasque-flower
A relaxing herb that will reduce the anxiety and occasional irrationality of these changes.

St John's Wort
Apart from its wide range of uses in many other bodily systems, this wonder-ful remedy is almost specific for depression and tension associated with the menopause.

Scullcap
A widely applicable relaxing remedy.

Valerian
A good herb where stronger sedating may be called for.

Drug Therapy

The usual result on going to the doctor for help with problems to do with anxiety or depression will be a prescription. It is unfortunate that the admirable British health service has become so pressured by the demands made on it that perhaps it should now be called the 'disease' service. Whilst the doctors and nurses are valiantly doing their best to help and care for their patients, the system has become so starved of funds that they cannot do what they would wish. The result in terms of 'nerve' conditions is that vast amounts of drugs are thrown at the problem.

As is shown throughout this book, such an approach is short-sighted and potentially dangerous. Where there are major psychological problems there can be no doubt that drug therapy has much to offer. In the treatment of schizophrenia and psychosis in general, great advances have been made through the use of drugs. However, the use of drugs in the treatment of the so-called 'neuroses', anxiety, etc., has masked the basic problems and unfortunately led to the development of new ones.

Anyone taking drugs for any psychological condition should know what they are being given and what side-effects may occur. If the drugs are being dropped, then the question of withdrawal effects arises. This chapter is a brief review of the commonly used drugs and their effects. The symptoms reviewed are those that medical experience has shown can occur. It does not mean that they will occur to you. Use this as a reference source.

The drugs referred to are those commonly used in anxiety, tension and its associated manifestations. No mention will be made of anti-depressant drugs or those used in the care of major psychological problems.

Sedatives and Hypnotics

A broad approach to help alleviate sleeplessness and sleep disturbance is discussed elsewhere in the book. This section is about the possible impact of the various drugs that are commonly available.

Sedatives and hypnotics are drugs that depress brain function. In small doses they are used as *sedatives* which calm and reduce tension, and in larger doses will induce sleep and are called *hypnotics*. All such drugs are potentially addictive and can quickly produce psychological dependence. The restless sleep that often follows the stopping of these drugs also strengthens the dependence. They are often unnecessary in the first place.

If taken regularly at a dose above that recommended they will cause intoxication. Even elderly and debilitated people, or people with heart, kidney or liver problems may develop intoxication at 'normal' dosage. The signs of such intoxication include confusion, difficulty in speaking, unsteadiness, poor memory, faulty judgement, irritability, overemotion, hostility, suspiciousness and even suicidal tendencies.

All drugs in this goup can produce physical dependence and resultant withdrawal symptoms if the drug is suddenly stopped. These may include anxiety, trembling, weakness, dizziness, nausea, vomiting, convulsions, delirium and – rarely – death. Compared to the number of people taking these drugs, physical dependence is rare, but psychological dependence is very common. Tolerance to the drugs is common and leads to less effect from the same dose over time. This carries the danger that the dose will be increased to obtain the same effect. If the dose is bring increased in this way there is a distinct chance of addiction.

All these drugs, and especially the barbiturates, can produce anxiety, irritability and depression, and since such drugs are often given to ease such symptoms in the first place there may be the temptation simply to give a higher dose. In some cases they may make things worse. There is some evidence that drug-induced sleep interferes with the normal restorative functions of sleep.

A sign of these possible problems is that the drug may help sleep and the person may awake feeling less tense,

only to become tired, irritable and bad-tempered later in the day. The drug may therefore impair learned behavious and the ability to concentrate.

There are a number of drugs that may be used.

BARBITURATES

These are amongst the oldest synthetic sedatives, and have been in use for almost a hundred years. They are used in the treatment of anxiety, tension and restlessness as well as sleep problems. The barbiturates used to produce sleep have an effect for about eight hours and all cause some degree of 'hangover'. There is a great risk of psychological and physiological dependence and they have been largely replaced by the benzodiazepines, which increase the action of alcohol and are a common agent in accidental or intentional overdose.

A large number of barbiturates are available on prescription and include: Phenobarbitone, Amytal, Sodium Amytal, Nembutal, Seconal, Hypnogen, Soneryl, Phanodorm.

NON-BARBITURATE HYPNOTICS

A diverse group of non-barbiturate drugs can be used to induce sleep. Many are rarely used now, such as bromide and chloral hydrate (a Mickey Finn). All the drugs in this group have the potential of producing tolerance and addiction, increase the effects of alcohol, interfere with the ability to concentrate and drive, and cause intoxication.

Examples of such drugs are: Welldorm. Quaalude, Mandrax, Oblivon.

ANTI-HISTAMINES

The anti-histamines, usually used for the suppression of allergy reactions, produce drowsiness as a side-effect. This is sometimes used to promote sleep. Mandrax was a combination of two drugs, one of which was an anti-histamine.

BENZODIAZEPINES

These are discussed in detail below. They are the most widely used anti-anxiety drugs and include Librium and Valium. Any of them at high dose will induce sleep, but two most often used for sleep are Mogadon and Dalmane.

Minor Tranquillizers

These drugs are used primarily to treat anxiety and tension. By far the most important group here are the benzodiazepines, also used for sleeping problems.

BENZODIAZEPINES

These are the most widely prescribed anti-anxiety drugs, used for anxiety, insomnia, muscular tension, convulsions, and withdrawal symptoms from other drugs. A host of adverse effects accompany their use. They can cause confusion and will interfere with the ability to concentrate and use machinery or drive safely. The common effects are drowsiness and lethargy. They may cause a fall in blood pressure and stimulate the appetite. Headaches may occur as well as dizziness and nausea. Sometimes excitement is caused, so instead of becoming calm the person may look and act as if drunk. They will increase the effects of alcohol. It is now clear that they may produce a form of physical dependence. Withdrawal can be a problem unless approached the right way. This is discussed elsewhere.

The benzodiazepines include, amongst many others, the following proprietary drugs: Librium, Valium, Serenid, Nobrium, Ativan, Dalman, Tranxene, Euhypnos.

Herbal Medicine and Benzodiazepine Dependence

(or: How to get off Valium.)

The herbalist is not the best suited practitioner to deal with the growing problem of drug abuse and dependency; however, plants have so much to offer in easing withdrawal from the benzodiazepines it is worth exploring the undoubted value of herbs and counselling in this context. We shall not concern ourselves with the disturbing 'street' use of these drugs, where doses of up to 500 mg of valium have been recorded to produce euphoria and intoxication.

It is unfortunately safe to assume that a very large number of people in this country are on long-term benzodiazepine use and so can be considered to be 'dependent'. Repeat prescribing of these drugs has serious social consequences, the most important of which are the effects on the individual. Long-term users may experience what has been called 'emotional anaesthesia' and a marked lowering of score in objective psychological tests. However, most long-term users no longer need such medication, the repeated prescribing occuring for many reasons other than the original need.

A dose in excess of 40 mg daily will, after three months, produce withdrawal symptoms if stopped, and some sensitive people will experience the same with smaller doses over a shorter period.

Someone wanting to stop using the drug may have been taking it for months or years and may have increased the dose to achieve the same effect. When it is abruptly discontinued, withdrawal symptoms may occur. This may range from anxiety and depression, through severe emotional and perceptive changes to (rarely) convulsions. The anxiety will be similar to that for which the drug was prescribed in the first place and so prompt the recommencement of treatment. The rather frightening symptoms that may occur include depression, insomnia, nausea, malaise and depersonalization, also perceptual changes such as shimmering lights, loud noises, unsteadiness and a sensation of motion.

The incidence and impact of such distressing withdrawal can be greatly alleviated by a step-wise reduction in dosage accompanied by the appropriate herbal medication as a bridge. Whilst this can be done on one's own, it is always best to get skilled and qualified herbal advice in this process.

WITHDRAWAL OF BENZODIAZEPINES

To do this effectively it is essential to know which type of benzodiazepine is being used. They can be divided into those that have active metabolites and therefore stay longer in the blood, and those that spend less time in the body because they don't have such metabolites. Thus:

Drugs with longer lasting action (the trade names of the drugs are given in brackets):
Chlordiazepoxide (Librium)
Diazepam (Valium)
Nitrazepam (Mogadon)
Flurazepam (Dalmane)
Clorazepate (Tranxene)
Shorter half-life:
Lorazepam (Activan)
Oxazepam (Serenid)
Temazepam (Euhypnos)

This differentiation is important not just for obvious therapeutic reasons, but because the mode of withdrawal is

Table 4: Main active metabolites in named drugs.

Drug	Half-life (hours)	Main active metabolite	Half-life (hours)	Speed of entry into brain
chlordiazepoxide	10–20	N-desmethyl-chlordiazepoxide	10–30	slow
diazepam	12–24	nordiazepam	50–90	fast
clorazepate	mainly hydrolysed before absorption	nordiazepam	50–90	slow
flurazepam	very short	N-desalkyl-flurazepam	50–100	medium
clobazam	10–30	N-desmethyl-clobazam	30–50	slow
nitrazepam	20–40	none		medium
lorazepam	10–20	none		slow
oxazepam	10–20	none		slow
temazepam	5–9	none		fast

(From: *Topics in Drug Therapy*, The Open University Press, 1982)

different for each group. First let's look at the orthodox approach for withdrawal followed by a herbal method.

It has been suggested that withdrawal is more severe and less successful in long-term users who are on a benzodiazepine with a short half-life. The withdrawal symptoms appear to be related to a rapid fall in blood levels of the drug. Table 4 shows how the main active metabolite affects the experienced activity of the ingested drug.

So the orthodox approach to weaning is based on a gradual reduction of dosage with a change of chosen drug at critical phases of the process. What is said here does not take into account the effect of age, disease or drug interactions on pharmacological activity.

1 *Patients on short half-life benzodiazepines*
    (a) A reduction by one-eighth every 2–4 weeks.
    (b) When lowest dose reached, *change* to lowest dose of long half-life benzodiazepine.
2 *Patients on long half-life benzodiazepines*
    (a) A reduction by one-eighth every 2–4 weeks.
    (b) Reach lowest therapeutic dose.
    (c) Further reduction every two weeks for 4–8 weeks. If physical symptoms arise add Propranolol (60–120 mg) or Oxypertine (10–20 mg) daily.
    (d) Stop benzodiazepines and reassess every four weeks.

From this it is clear that the process takes a long time. However the whole process can be speeded up safely by using herbal remedies at the same time. Not only will this reduce withdrawal symptoms, more importantly it will tone and strengthen the nervous system after its exposure to intense chemical stress (paradoxically meant to relieve the psychological impact of life stress!).

HERBS AND WITHDRAWAL

With the range of herbal remedies available to us it is possible to ease the weaning process whilst treating for specific bodily symptoms if they arise. It cannot be stressed enough that the aim is to help the person come off drugs and the need for an artificial psychological support, *not* to replace benzodiazepines with herbal nervines. This is, unfortunately, too easy to do.

The whole of the individual's health and well-being must be seen to at the same time, as the tranquillizers will have had a traumatic effect upon the whole system. The advice given here is for the nervous system itself, and, of course, the unique situation in each person of liver, kidneys, digestion, etc. must be supported. This is where a qualified medical herbalist will help.

As each person is so unique it is impossible to give doses and specific prescriptions. The herbs mentioned below should be studied in the herbal section of the book to find which will be most appropriate in each case. However, the following remedies could act as the core of such a process: Scullcap and Valerian.

To these may be added other nervines, bitters, tonic herbs, etc. Bitters, such as Wormwood and Mugwort, will aid the whole system regain tone and vitality. This happens through a toning action on the digestive and endocrine systems. The health of the liver must be supported because of its vital de-toxifying role. Golden Seal and Dandelion Root would be worth considering.

Any specific physical symptom can be treated by the appropriate herbs. For example, Motherwort if there are heart palpitations, Comfrey or Marshmallow Root for stomach ulcers. It would be worth reading the section on physical symptoms on page 19. It is difficult to generalize too freely, as different people will have different herbs indicated. Ones that I have found useful on occasions are: Motherwort; Pasque-flower; Oats;

Lavender; St John's Wort; Passion-flower.

This is just a partial list of favourite remedies which may well be different for each herbalist. The dosage levels and times do not appear to be critical – a dose three times a day suits some whilst the total daily dosage at once helps others. A regular dose supplemented by extra doses when the person feels the need appears to be most effective. However, the dosage is very variable, with some people being very sensitive to herbs such as Scullcap, whilst others may need much more. The actual withdrawal procedure may be as follows:

2–4 days on drugs plus the herbs
4–5 days dropping one-sixth of the drug dose plus herbs;
4–5 days for each subsequent sixth of the drug dose. Increase herbal dosage

if needed and specific herbal help with any bodily symptoms.

The process can be quicker than this or longer. Do not try to go too fast, because if a feeling of failure develops it compounds the whole operation. Constant reassurance and support are vital, especially from close family and work colleagues.

Supportive counselling and a willingness to help in gaining insights from any psychological patterns that appear during the process helps. Sometimes active in-depth psychotherapy is useful, but this should only be started if the person is feeling physically strong and able. Usually, however, there is more than enough going on anyway.

A good, healthy and balanced diet is essential, with a possible need for supplements of the B complex vitamins and vitamin C.

How to Use Herbs

There are a multitude of ways to use and prepare herbal remedies. Here we shall focus on the ways that will aid the relaxation process most effectively. Ways of preparing ointments, poultices and suppositories will not be explained here as they rarely come into stress and tension relief. If you do want to know more about these, any of the herbals mentioned in the bibliography will give recipes and ideas.

Fresh Herbs

It is almost always preferable to use herbs freshly picked, as they will be rich in essential oils and also still full of life. Some herbs are delicious additions to the dinner table but if you choose to eat your medicine this way, these modern times necessitate careful field identification as well as non-polluted gathering places. For example, roadside dandelions do not make healthy salads! It would be far better to combine a restful country walk with the collection of a few wild plants. Have respect and care, not only to pick the right plant but also to pick only the amounts you need at that time.

If you have a juicer, some fresh plants can yield their live-healing energy and constituents this way, but it is necessary to drink the juice quickly or much of its energy is easily oxidized and lost. Of course, this is not always possible, in which case dried herbs or tinctures will do. The few exceptions are those plants that contain potentially dangerous natural chemicals that change to become quite safe on drying. The best example here is Pasque-flower which should never be used fresh but is perfectly safe when dried. Guidance on this is always given in herbals.

As a very rough guide, a handful of fresh leaves is equivalent to a teaspoonful of the dried herb. This approximation is useful, as most dosages are given for dried herbs or tinctures.

Infusion should be made in the same way as described for dried herbs, ensuring the teapot is covered so that a minimum of essential aromatic oil is lost. If you can smell your fresh Peppermint tea two rooms away, then most of the oil has been lost!

Dried Herbs

A large range of dried medicinal herbs is available these days. As long as they are bought from a reputable company you can be sure of their quality due to the work of the British Herbal Medicine Association. It is important for the importers and packers to know that the cut, dried leaf is what the label says it is. The main companies have professional pharmacognosticists working for them, checking all the herbs.

The dosage of each herb varies and the details of specific levels is given in the herbal, but as most of the remedies suggested in this book are quite safe, general guidelines can be given without fear of an overdose. However, always check in a herbal before using an unfamiliar herb.

If a remedy consists of leaves, petals, fruits or even a root rich in aromatic oils, the tea should be made as an *infusion*. If it is woody, a root, bark or a rhizome, then a *decoction* should be prepared.

Infusion

Pour 1 pint (0.5 litre) of boiling water onto 1 oz (25 g) of finely chopped dried herb in a warmed pot. Cover and let steep for 10–15 minutes. Strain and then keep in a covered container.

Decoction

Add 1 oz (25 g) of chopped herb to 1 pint (0.5 litre) of cold water, bring to the boil and gently simmer for 10–15 minutes. Let cool, strain and then keep in a covered container.

DOSAGE

Always check in a herbal that the dose you are taking is the correct one, but for the vast majority of herbs the following is fine. Take one wineglass of the infusion or decoction three times a day. In most cases, a regular dose every eight hours is the most effective. Of course, with a sleeping mixture this would be quite different as it is taken at night, the dosage depending on the sensitivity of the person involved. Experiment until you and the herbs are familiar with each other, and the dosage is satisfactorily effective. This is quite safe! The tea should usually be taken between meals. A wineglassful is about the same as three tablespoonsful.

The dose should be reduced for the young and old. Thus it should be halved at the ages 70–75 or ten.

Teas made in this way will keep for three to four days if kept covered in a refrigerator. If this is not possible, then they should be made fresh each day.

TINCTURES

An increasingly popular way of taking herbs is in the form of a water/alcohol extract called a tincture, which is very concentrated and makes it easy to compound medicines. However, it makes the dosage calculations complex and so they are best used under the guidance of a skilled medical herbalist.

BATHS

A pleasant way to use relaxing herbs is in the form of a bath. Here the tea or extract is added to a hot bath. The whole pint of an infusion or decoction described above would be appropriate for an adult. Another way to prepare a bath would be for the herbs to be wrapped in a muslin or cheesecloth bag and hung under the hot-water tap. When the water is run it turns the bath into an infusion. Any herb can be used in this way, but the aromatic relaxing remedies are best.

OILS

Essential oils are used in a quite different way to straight herbal remedies and are described in the section on aromatherapy. They make wonderful baths, too.

Herbal Actions

In the herbal that follows, each herb is described in the same format, and includes a list of the 'Actions' of that remedy.

An action is one of the medical attributes of the herb, and it tells us how the plant may work on the body. Many diferent plants can have actions in common, and an understanding of what they mean provides a way of prescribing that greatly aids the work of the medical herbalist. They can be explored further in some of the herbals suggested in the bibliography.

Some of the actions have rather outlandish names, so here is a selected list of definitions. It is only a partial list that covers points raised in this book; a complete list is unnecessary:

Alternative: Herbs that will gradually restore the proper functioning of the body and restore health. They are the old-fashioned 'blood cleansers'.

Analgesic Anodyne: Pain reliever.

Anti-catarrhal: Herbs that get rid of excess catarrh from the body.

Anti-inflammatory: Remedies that reduce the inflammatory response in the body. They may be used internally or externally. These herbs are not suppressants in the way that steroid drugs may be.

Expectorant: Will clear phlegm from the lungs.

Hypnotic: Herbs that induce sleep, not a hypnotic trance!

Laxative: Promote the evacuation of the bowels.

Nervine: Remedies that effect the nervous system, usually toning and strengthening. There are subdivisions of this action that are discussed in the book.

Sedative: Plants that calm the nervous system, reducing anxiety and tension throughout the body. Herbal sedatives in this book are not addictive.

Stimulant: Quicken and enliven the physiological functioning of the body. Whole herbs usually give optimum activity rather than artificially inducing 'hyped-up' activity.

Tonic: Herbs that strengthen and enliven either specific organs or the whole body.

Vulnerary: Plants that aid and speed the healing of cuts and wounds.

Herbal

This is by no means a complete list of herbal remedies that can be used in the treatment of stress-related problems. I have left out plants that are on the scheduled drugs list or poisonous at certain dosage levels, as well as some of the less commonly used ones such as Asafoetida.

BETONY (Wood Betony)
(Betonica officinalis (Stachys betonica), Labiatae)

Part used—dried aerial parts

Collection—the aerial parts should be collected just before the flowers bloom. They should be dried carefully in the sun.

Actions—relaxant, sedative, a gentle stimulant of circulation to the head, nervine tonic, digestive bitter.

Indications—Betony feeds and strengthens the central nervous system whilst also having a sedative action upon the mind and 'nerves' in general. It finds use in *nervous debility* where this is associated with *anxiety* and *tension*. It will ease headaches and neuralgia when they are of nervous origin. Betony can help in sinus catarrh or other forms of catarrhal congestion in the head. Because of its bitter nature it aids poor digestion due to debility.

Combinations—for the treatment of *nervous headache* it combines well with Scullcap, Lime Blossom and Lavender Flowers.

Dosage—1–4 g (about 1–2 teaspoonsful) of the dried herb in an infusion three times a day.

BLACK COHOSH
(Cimicifuga racemosa, Ranunculaceae)

Part used—root and rhizome.

Collection—the roots are unearthed with the rhizome in autumn after the fruits have ripened. They should be cut lengthwise and dried carefully.

Actions—emmenagogue, antispasmodic, alternative sedative, vasodilator, diaphoretic.

Indications—Black Cohosh is a most valuable herb that comes to us via the North American Indians. It has a powerful action as a relaxant and a normalizer of the female reproductive system, and so may be used beneficially in cases of *painful* or *delayed menstruation*. *Ovarian cramps* or *cramping pain* in the womb will be relieved by Black Cohosh. It has a normalizing action on the balance of female sex hormones and may safely be used to regain normal hormonal activity. It is very active in the treatment of *rheumatic pains*, but also in *rheumatoid arthritis, osteo-arthritis*, in *muscular* and *neurological pain*. It finds use in *sciatica* and *neuralgia*. As a relaxing nervine it may be used in many situations where such an agent is needed. Black Cohosh will reduce spasm and so aid in the treatment of pulmonary complaints such as *whooping cough*. It has been found beneficial in cases of *tinnitus*.

Combinations—for uterine conditions combine with Blue Cohosh. For rheumatic problems use with Bogbean.

Caution—High doses of this plant may cause dizziness and agitation in sensitive people. It should not be used in pregnancy.

Dosage—0.2–1 g of the dried rhizome three times a day, decocted as a tea or tincture.

BLACK HAW
(Viburnum prunifolium, Caprifoliaciae)

Part used—dried bark of root or stem.

Collection—the bark from the roots and the trunk is collected in the autumn. The shrubs should be dug out and the bark stripped from roots and trunk. The bark from branches should be collected in spring and summer. In both cases the bark should be dried in the shade.

Actions—anti-spasmodic, sedative, hypotensive, astringent.

Indications—Black Haw has a very similar use to Cramp-bark, to which it is closely related. It is a powerful relaxant of the uterus and is used for *dysmenorrhoea* (uterine cramps or period pains) and *false labour pains*. It may be used in *threatened miscarriage* as well. Its relaxant and sedative actions explain its power in reducing *blood pressure*, which happens through a relaxation of the peripheral blood vessels. Black Haw also has a reputation in the treatment of *vaginal* and *cervical discharges*. It may be used as a general anti-spasmodic in the treatment of *asthma*.

Combinations—for threatened miscarriage it will combine well with False Unicorn Root and Cramp-bark.

Dosage—2–4 g (1–2 teaspoonsful) of dried bark decocted three times a day as a tea or as tincture.

BLACK HOREHOUND
(Ballota nigra, Labiatae)

Part used—dried aerial parts.

Collection—the herb should be gathered just as it begins to bloom in July.

Actions—anti-emetic, sedative, mild astringent, emmenagogue, expectorant.

Indications—Black Horehound – which should not be confused with White Horehound – is an excellent remedy for the settling of *nausea* and *vomiting* where the cause lies within the nervous system rather than in the stomach. It may be used with safety in *motion sickness*, for example, where the nausea is triggered through the inner ear and the central nervous system. This herb will also be of value in helping the *vomiting of pregnancy* or nausea and vomiting due to nervousness. This remedy has a reputation as a normalizer of *menstrual function* and also as a mild expectorant.

Combinations—for the relief of nausea and vomiting it may be combined with Meadow-sweet, Chamomile or Peppermint.

Dosage—1–4 g (1–2 teaspoonsful) of the dried herb infused as a tea or in the form of tincture.

BLUE COHOSH

(*Caulophyllum thalictroides*, Berberidaceae)

Part used—rhizome and root.

Collection—the roots and rhizome are collected in the autumn, as at the end of the growing season they are richest in natural chemicals.

Actions—uterine tonic, emmenagogue, anti-spasmodic, anti-rheumatic.

Indications—Blue Cohosh is a plant that comes to us from the North American Indians, which shows in its other names of *Squaw Root* and *Papoose Root*. It is an excellent *uterine* and *fallopian tube tonic* that may be used in any situation where there is a weakness or loss of tone. It may be used at any time during pregnancy if there is a threat of miscarriage. Similarly, because of its anti-spasmodic action, it will ease *false labour pains*. However, when labour does ensue, the use of Blue Cohosh just before birth will help ensure an easy delivery. In all these cases it is a safe herb to use. As an emmenagogue it can be used to bring on a *delayed* or *suppressed menstruation* whilst ensuring that the pain that sometimes accompanies it is relieved. It will alleviate the pains that may accompany any *pelvic inflammation* or even *fibroids*. Blue Cohosh may be used in cases where an anti-spasmodic is needed, such as in *colic*, *asthma* or *nervous coughs*. It has a reputation for easing *rheumatic pain*.

Combinations—to strengthen the uterus it could be used with False Unicorn Root, Motherwort and Yarrow.

Dosage—0.2–1 g of dried rhizome decocted as a tea, or its equivalent in tincture, three times a day.

BUGLEWEED

(*Lycopus europaeus*, Labiatae)

Common name—Water Horehound.

Part used—aerial parts.

Collection—it should be collected just before the buds open.

Actions—cardioactive diuretic, peripheral vasoconstrictor, astringent, sedative, thryroxine antagonist, antitussive.

Indications—Bugleweed is a specific for *over-active thyroid glands*, especially where the symptoms include tightness of breathing, and palpitations that are of nervous origin. Bugleweed will aid the *weak heart* where there is associated *build-up of water* in the body. As a sedative cough reliever it will ease *irritating coughs*, especially when they are of nervous origin. Such problems should, however, be diagnosed and treated by a qualified practitioner.

Combinations—Bugleweed may be used with nervines such as Scullcap or Valerian.

Dosage—1–2 g of the dried herb infused as a tea, or its equivalent in tincture form.

CALIFORNIAN POPPY

(*Eschscholzia californica*, Papaveraceae)

Part used—dried aerial parts.

Collection—the aerial parts are collected at the time of flowering which is between June and September. They should be dried in the shade.

Actions—Sedative, hypnotic, anti-spasmodic, anodyne.

Indications—Californian Poppy has the reputation of being a non-addictive alternative to the Opium Poppy, though it is less powerful. It has been used as a sedative and hypnotic for children, where there is *over-excitability* and *sleeplessness*. It can be used wherever an anti-spasmodic remedy is required. The American Indians used it for *colic pains* and it may be useful in the treatment of *gall-bladder colic*.

Dosage—2–4 g of the dried herb infused as a tea should be drunk at night to promote restful sleep.

CHAMOMILE, GERMAN
(*Matricaria chamomilla*, Compositae)

Part used—the flowers.

Collection—the flowers should be gathered between May and August when they are not wet with dew or rain. They should be dried with care at not too high a temperature.

Actions—relaxant, anti-spasmodic, carminative, anti-inflammatory, analgesic, antiseptic, vulnerary.

Indications—Chamomile is renowned for its medical and household uses. The aparently endless list of conditions it can help all fall into areas that the relaxing, carminative and anti-inflammatory actions can aid. It is an excellent, gentle sedative, useful and safe for use with children. It will contribute its relaxing actions in any combinations and is thus used in *anxiety* and *insomnia*. Indigestion and *inflammations* such as *gastritis* are often eased with Chamomile. Similarly, it can be used as a mouthwash for inflammations of the mouth such as *gingivitis* and for bathing *inflamed and sore eyes*. As a gargle it will help *sore throats*. As an inhalation over a steam bath, it will speed recovery from *nasal catarrh*. Externally, it will speed *wound healing* and reduce the swelling due to *inflammation*. As a carminative with relaxing properties it will ease *flatulence* and *dyspeptic pain*.

Dosage—1–4 g of the flower heads (1–2 teaspoonsful) infused as a tea, or its tincture equivalent, taken three times a day or more. This tea can act as a wash for external use.

COWSLIP
(*Primula veris*, Primulaceae)

Part used—the yellow petals and the root.

Collection—the flower corollae should be gathered without the green calyx, between March and May. Dry quickly in the shade. The roots should be unearthed either before Cowslip flowers or in the autumn. Over-collecting has led to this beautiful plant becoming increasingly rare. Only pick if present in abundance and then only pick limited amounts.

Actions—flowers: sedative, anti-spasmodic; root: expectorant.

Indications—Cowslip is an excellent, generally applicable relaxing, sedative remedy. It will ease reactions to *stress* and *tension*, relaxing nervous excitement and facilitating restful sleep. It may be used with safety in *bronchitis, colds, chills* and *congestive coughs*. It has been used as part of a broad treatment of *whooping cough*. Try it in *nervous headaches* and *insomnia*.

Combinations—For *stress-related problems* it may be used with any of the relaxing nervines such as Lime Blossom or Scullcap. For *coughs* it may be used with Coltsfoot, White Horehound and Aniseed.

Dosage—1–4 g of the dried flowers (about 1–2 teaspoonsful) as an infused tea three times a day for anxiety or at night to aid sleep.

CRAMP-BARK

(*Viburnum opulus*, Caprifoliacea)
Part used—dried bark.
Collection—the bark is collected in April and May, cut into pieces and dried.
Actions—anti-spasmodic, sedative, relaxant to smooth muscle, astringent.
Indications—Cramp-bark shows by its name the richly deserved reputation it has as a relaxer of *muscular tension* and *spasm*. It has two main areas of use: firstly, in *muscular cramps* and, secondly, in *ovarian* and *uterine muscle problems*. Cramp-bark will relax the uterus and so relieve painful cramps associated with periods (*dysmenorrhoea*). In a similar way it may be used to protect from *threatened miscarriage*. Cramp-bark will ease *colicky pain* in the gut, gall-bladder and urinary system. Some cases of *migraine* and other conditions due to *muscle spasm* will be eased. In conjunction with other remedies it may help in the reduction of *raised blood pressure*. It has been used to help quieten overactive or convulsive states in children. Its astringent action gives it a role in the treatment of *excessive blood loss in periods* and especially *bleeding associated with the menopause*.
Combinations—for the relief of *cramp* it may be combined with Prickly Ash and Wild Yam. For *uterine* and *ovarian pains* or *threatened miscarriage* it may be

used with Black Haw and Valerian.
Dosage—1–4 g of the bark made into a decoction and drunk three times a day. The tincture alternative can be used.

DAMIANA

(*Turnera aphrodisiaca*, Turneraceae)
Part used—dried leaves and stems.
Collection—the leaves and stems are gathered at the time of flowering.
Actions—nerve tonic, anti-depressant, urinary antiseptic, mildly laxative.
Indications—Damiana is an excellent strengthening remedy for the nervous system. It has an ancient reputation as an aphrodisiac. Whilst this may or may not be true, it has a definite tonic action on the central nervous and the hormonal system. The pharmacology of the plant suggests that the alkaloids could have a testosterone-like action (testosterone is a male hormone). As a useful anti-depressant, Damiana is considered to be a specific in cases of *anxiety* and *depression* where there is a sexual factor. It may be used to strengthen the male sexual system.
Combinations—as a nerve tonic it is often used with Oats. Depending on the situation it combines well with Kola or Scullcap.
Dosage—1–4 g of the herb or its equivalent as an infusion three times a day. The tincture equivalent may be used.

FEVERFEW

(*Tanacetum parthenium*, Compositae)
Part used—leaves.
Collection—the leaves may be picked throughout the spring and summer,

although just before flowering is best.

Actions—anti-inflammatory, vasodilatory, relaxant, digestive bitter, uterine stimulant.

Indications—Feverfew has regained its deserved reputation as a primary remedy in the treatment of *migraine headaches*, especially those that are relieved by applying warmth to the head. It may also help *arthritis* when it is in the painfully active inflammatory stage. *Dizziness* and *tinnitus* may be eased, especially if used in conjunction with other remedies. *Painful periods* and sluggish menstrual flow will be relieved by Feverfew.

Caution—Feverfew should not be used during pregnancy because of the stimulant action on the womb. The fresh leaves may cause mouth ulcers in sensitive people.

Dosage—it is best to use the equivalent of one fresh leaf for 1–3 times a day. It is best used fresh or frozen.

GINSENG
(Panax ginseng, Araliaceae)

Part used—root.

Collection—Ginseng is cultivated in China, Korea and N. E. America (Panax quinquefolium).

Actions—anti-depressive, increases resistance and improves both physical and mental performance, adaptogen.

Indications—Ginseng has an ancient history and as such has accumulated much folklore about its actions and uses. Many of the claims that surround it are inflated, but it is clear that this is a unique plant. It has a direct action on the adrenal cortex by improving its responses to stress. Ginseng has the power to move a person to their physical peak, and is especially helpful for debility,

degenerative conditions and problems of *old age*. In the short term it will improve stamina and concentration, aid healing and increase resistance to *stress* generally. It will raise *lowered blood pressure* to a normal level, and ease *depression*, especially where this is due to debility and exhaustion. It can be used in general for *exhaustion states* and *weakness*. It has a reputation as an aphrodisiac.

Caution—should not be used over extensive periods of time, or if headaches start after using the herb. To be avoided in high blood pressure.

Dosage—for treatment of debility or to aid the elderly, use 400–800 mg of the root a day. For short-term treatment of stress use 600–2000 mg of the dried root or its equivalent each day for up to three weeks.
(See **Siberian Ginseng.**)

GOLDENROD
(Solidago virgaurea, Compositae)

Part used—aerial parts.

Actions—anti-inflammatory, anti-catarrhal, urinary antiseptic, relaxant.

Indications—whilst primarily used as an excellent herb for relieving *upper respiratory catarrh*, it will also help where such problems are compounded by *nervous tension* and *restlessness*.

Dosage—0.5–2 g (about 1 teaspoonful) of the dried herb made into an infused tea three times a day.

GOTU KOLA
(Hydrocotyle asiatica, Umbelliferae)

Part used—leaves and stems.

Actions—relaxant, nervine tonic,

digestive bitter, diuretic, anti-inflammatory, vulnerary.

Indications—this tropical plant has a growing reputation in Britain as a restorative, relaxing remedy for the nervous system. It may be of help in a whole range of neurological and mental disturbances, especially *stress-related debility*. It may be used in inflammatory diseases such as *rheumatism*. In the East, Gotu Kola has a good reputation for the treatment of poorly healing wounds and ulcers.

Dosage—0.5–2 g of the dried herb (about 1 teaspoonful) infused as a tea taken three times a day.

HOPS
(Humulus lupulus, Cannabinaceae)
Part used—flower inflorescence.

Collection—the Hops cones are gathered before they are fully ripe in August and September. They should be dried with care in the shade.

Actions—sedative, hypnotic, antiseptic, astringent, bitter.

Indications—Hops is a remedy that has a marked relaxing effect upon the central nervous sytem. It is used extensively for the treatment of *insomnia*. It will ease *tension* and *anxiety*, and may be used where this tensions leads to *restlessness, headache* and possibly *indigestion*. As an stringent with these relaxing properties it can be used in conditions such as *mucous colitis*. It should, however, be avoided where there is a marked degree of depression as this may be accentuated. Externally the antiseptic action is utilized for the treatment of *ulcers*.

Caution—do not use in cases with marked depression.

Combinations—for *insomnia* it can be combined with Valerian and Passion-flower.

Dosage—0.5–1 g (about a teaspoonful) of the flowers as an infused tea three times a day. A much stronger tea may be used at night to promote sleep.

HYSSOP
(Hyssopus officinalis, Labiatae)
Part used—dried aerial parts.

Collection—the flowering tops of Hyssop should be collected in August and dried in the sun.

Actions—anti-spasmodic, expectorant, diaphoretic, sedative, carminative.

Indications—Hyssop has an interesting range of uses which are largely attributable to the anti-spasmodic action of the volatile oil. It is used in *coughs, bronchitis* and *chronic catarrh*. Its diaphoretic properties explain its use in the *common cold*. As a nervine it may be used in *anxiety states, hysteria* and *petit mal* (a form of epilepsy).

Combinations—it may be combined with White Horehound and Coltsfoot in the treatment of *coughs* and *bronchitis*. For the *common cold* it may be mixed with Boneset, Elder Flower and Peppermint.

Dosage—1–4 g (1–2 teaspoonsful) of the dried herb infused as a tea three times a day.

JAMAICAN DOGWOOD
(Piscidia erythrina, Leguminosae)
Part used—stem bark.

Collection—the bark is collected in vertical strips from trees growing in the Caribbean, Mexico and Texas.

Actions—sedative, anodyne.

Indications—Jamaican Dogwood is a powerful sedative, used in its West Indian homeland as a fish poison. Whilst not being poisonous to humans, the given dosage level should not be exceeded. It is a powerful remedy for the treatment of painful conditions such as *neuralgia* and *migraine*. It can also be used in the relief of *ovarian* and *uterine pain*. Its main use is perhaps in *insomnia* where this is related to nervous tension or pain. It may be found helpful in some cases of migraine.

Combinations—for the easing of *insomnia* it is best combined with Hops and Valerian. For *dysmenorrhoea (painful periods)* it may be used with Black Haw.

Dosage—0.5–2 g (a teaspoonful) of the dried bark made into a tea as a decoction taken three times a day. The tincture may be used as well.

KAVA KAVA
(Piper methysticum, Piperaceae)

Part used—rhizome.

Actions—urinary antiseptic and diuretic, circulatory stimulant, antispasmodic, psychoactive.

Indications—This exotic herb from the South Pacific has its main use in the treatment of urinary infection. It can be used in small dosage as a mental stimulant, but at higher dosage it will slow down mental awareness. In its native lands the fresh plant has been prepared to produce an active psychedelic product.

Dosage—1–4 g of the rhizome as a decoction three times a day.

KOLA
(Cola vera, Sterculiaceae)

Part used—seed kernel.

Collection—the Kola tree grows in tropical Africa and is cultivated in South America. The seeds are collected when ripe and are initially white, turning the characteristic red upon drying.

Actions—stimulant to central nervous system, anti-depressive, astringent, diuretic.

Indications—Kola has a marked stimulating effect on human consciousness. It can be used wherever there is a need for direct stimulation, which is less often than is usually thought. Through regaining proper health and therefore right functioning, the nervous system does not need such help. In the short term it may be used for *nervous debility*, in states of *atony* and *weakness*. It can act as a specific in *nervous diarrhoea*. It will aid in states of *depression* and may in some people give rise to euphoric states. In some varieties of *migraine* it can help greatly. Through the stimulation it will be a valuable part of the treatment for *anorexia*. It can be viewed as specific in cases of depression associated with weakness and debility.

Combinations—Kola will go well with Oats, Damiana, and scullcap.

Dosage—0.5–3 g (about 1–2 teaspoonsful) of the powdered seeds three times a day. The tincture may be used.

LADY'S-SLIPPER
(Cypripripedium pubescens, Orchidaceae)

Part used—the root.

Collection—Lady's-slipper is a protected plant in the United Kingdom and so should never be collected if found wild.

Actions—sedative, hypnotic, antispasmodic, nervine tonic.

Indications—Lady's-slipper is one of the most widely applicable nervines that we possess in the materia medica. It may be used in all *stress reactions, emotional tension* and *anxiety states*. It will help elevate the mood, especially where *depression* is present. It can help in easing *nervous pain*, though it is best used in combination with other herbs for this purpose. It is perhaps at its best when treating *anxiety* that is associated with *insomnia*.

Combinations—it combines well with Oats and Scullcap. For *nerve pain* it may be used with Jamaican Dogwood, Passion-flower and Valerian.

Dosage—1–4 g (1–2 teaspoonsful) of the dried root made into an infused tea, taken three times a day. A stronger cup can be drunk at night. This root is made into an infusion rather than a decoction because it is so rich in volatile oil. The tincture may be used.

LAVENDER
(*Lavendula officinalis*, Labiatae)
Part used—flowers.

Collection—the flowers should be gathered just before opening between June and September. They should be dried gently at a temperature not above 35°C.

Actions—Carminative, antispasmodic, anti-depressant, rubefacient.

Indications—this beautiful herb has many uses, culinary, cosmetic and medicinal. It is an effective herb for *headaches*, especially when they are related to stress. Lavender can be quite effective in the raising of *depression*, especially if used in conjunction with other remedies. As a gentle strengthening tonic of the nervous system it may be used in states of *nervous debility* and *exhaustion*. It can be used to soothe and promote natural sleep. Because of the carminative oil, Lavender will ease *digestive colic* and *flatulent dyspepsia*. Externally the oil is used as a stimulating liniment to help ease the aches and pains of *rheumatism* and *migraine*.

Combinations—for *depression* it will combine well with Rosemary, Kola, Damiana or Scullcap. For *headaches* it may be used with Lady's-slipper or Valerian.

Dosage—an infusion of fresh or dried flowers is made with 1–4 g (1–2 teaspoonsful), taking care to cover so that the aroma is not lost. Take three times a day.

LEMON BALM
(*Melissa officinalis*, Labiatae)
Part used—aerial parts.

Collection—the plant should be collected just before the flower blossoms open in midsummer. They should be collected on a dry day and dried carefully in the shade.

Actions—relaxant, carminative.

Indications—this useful herb can be used with equal value for tension affecting the nervous system and digestive system. It is widely applicable for all varieties of *anxiety* and *tension* related problems. It has particular relevance for childhood problems such as *overactivity*. It will ease many *indigestion* symptoms. Has been used in high dosage to treat *shingles*.

Dosage—1–4 g (1–2 teaspoonsful) of the dried herb infused as a tea three times a day, or as required.

LIFE ROOT
(*Senecio aureus*, Compositae)

Part used—aerial parts.

Actions—uterine relaxant and tonic, relaxant.

Indications—a wonderful remedy for gynaecological conditions, especially *menopausal problems*. Almost a specific for the emotional upset of the menopause. This herb should not be used during pregnancy.

Dosage—1–4 g (1–2 teaspoonsful of the dried herb infused as a tea three times a day.

LIME BLOSSOM (LINDEN)
(*Tilia europaea*, Tiliaceae)

Part used—dried flowers.

Collection—the flowers should be gathered immediately after flowering in the midsummer. They should be collected on a dry day and dried carefully in the shade.

Actions—nervine, anti-spasmodic, diaphoretic, diuretic, mild astringent.

Indications—Lime Blossom is well known as a relaxing remedy for use in *nervous tension*. It has a reputation as a prophylactic against the development of arteriosclerosis and hypertension. It is considered to be a specific in the treatment of raised blood pressure associated with arteriosclerosis and nervous tension. Its relaxing action combined with a general effect upon the circulatory system give Lime Blossom a role in the treatment of some forms of *migraine*. The diaphoresis combined with the relaxation explain its value in *feverish colds* and 'flu.

Combinations—in *raised blood pressure* it may be used with Hawthorn and Mistletoe, with Hops in nervous tension and with Elder Flower in the *common cold*.

Dosage—1–4 g (1–2 teaspoonsful) of the dried flowers infused as a tea three times a day. A stronger tea may be used at night.

LOBELIA
(*Lobelia inflata*, Campanulaceae)

Part used—aerial parts.

Collection—the entire plant above ground should be collected at the end of the flowering time, between August and September. The seed pods should be collected as well.

Actions—respiratory stimulant, anti-asthmatic, anti-spasmodic, expectorant, emetic.

Indications—Lobelia is one of the most useful systemic relaxants available to us. It has a general depressant action on the central and autonomic nervous system and on neuro-muscular action. It may be used in many conditions in combination with other herbs to further their effectiveness if relaxation is needed. Its primary specific use is in *bronchitic asthma* and *bronchitis*. An analysis of the action of the alkaloids present reveal apparently paradoxical effects. Lobeline is a powerful respiratory stimulant, whilst isolobinine is an emetic and respiratory relaxant, which will stimulate catarrhal secretion and expectoration whilst relaxing the muscles of the respiratory system. The overall action is a truly holistic combination of stimulation and relaxation! It plays a role in a holistic treatment of *allergic, inflammatory* and *hypersensitivity* reactions. It can be used externally to ease *muscle spasms*.

Combinations—It will combine well with Cayenne, Grindelia, Pill-bearing Spurge, Sundew and Ephedra in the treatment of *asthma*.

Dosage—As a dried herb this remedy should be used under the supervision of a qualified herbalist.

MATE
(Ilex paraguariensis, Aquifoliaceae)
Part used—leaves.

Actions—central nervous system stimulant, anti-spasmodic, diuretic.

Indications—Mate is used in South America in the way tea is used in Britain. Medically it helps with nervous headaches associated with fatigue. It may help control excessive appetite (if you're lucky!)

Caution—as with other caffeine-rich herbs such as tea and coffee, it should be drunk in moderation.

Dosage—1–2 g (a teaspoonful) of the dried leaves as an infusion drunk when wanted.

MISTLETOE
(Viscum album, Lorantheaceae)
Part used—the dried leafy twigs.

Collection—the young leafy twigs should be collected in the spring.

Actions—nervine, hypotensive, cardiac depressant, possible anti-tumour.

Indications—Mistletoe is an excellent relaxing nervine indicated in many cases. It will quieten, soothe and tone the nervous system. This remedy acts directly on the vagus nerve to reduce heart rate whilst strengthening the wall of the peripheral capillaries. It will thus act to reduce blood pressure and ease *arterio-sclerosis*. Where there is *nervous quickening of the heart (nervous tachycardia)* it may be very helpful. *Headache* due to high blood pressure is relieved by it. It has been shown by current cancer research to have some anti-tumour activity.

Combinations—it combines well with Hawthorn Berries and Lime Blossom in the treatment of *raised blood pressure*.

Caution—DO NOT USE THE BERRIES.

Dosage—1–2 g of the dried leaves as an infusion up to three times a day.

MOTHERWORT
(Leonurus cardiaca, Labiatae)
Part used—Aerial parts.

Collection—the stalks should be gathered at the time of flowering, which is between June and September.

Actions—sedative, emmenagogue, anti-spasmodic, uterine tonic, cardiac tonic, carminative.

Indications—the names of this plant show its range of uses. 'Motherwort' shows its relevance to menstrual and uterine conditions whilst 'cardiaca' indicates its use in heart and circulation treatments. It is valuable in the stimulation of *delayed* or *suppressed menstruation*, especially where there is anxiety or tension involved. It is a useful relaxing tonic for aiding in *menopausal changes*. It may be used to ease *false labour pains*. *Disturbance of menstrual cycles* due to tension and worry will be eased by this herb. It is an excellent tonic for the heart, strengthening without straining. It is a specific for *over-rapid heartbeat* where it is brought about by anxiety and other such causes. It may be used in all *heart conditions* that are associated with anxiety and tension.

Dosage—1–4g (1–2 teaspoonsful) of the dried herb as an infused tea or as the tincture.

MUGWORT

(Artemisia vulgaris, Compositae)

Part used—leaves or root

Collection—the leaves and flowering stalks should be gathered just at blossoming time, which is between July and September.

Actions—bitter tonic, stimulant, nervine tonic, emmenagogue.

Indications—Mugwort can be used wherever a digestive stimulant is called for. It will aid the digestion through the bitter stimulation of the juices whilst also providing a carminative oil. It has a mildly nervine action in aiding *depression* and easing *tension*, which appears to be due to the bolatile oil, so it is essential that this is not lost in preparation. Mugwort may also be used as an emmenagogue in the aiding of *normal menstrual flow.*

Dosage—0.5–2 g (1 teaspoonful) of the dried herb used as an infused tea three times a day. The tincture may be used.

OATS

(Avena sativa, Gramineae)

Part used—seeds and the whole plant.

Collection—the fruit and straw are gathered at harvest time, in August about four weeks after the rye harvest. The stalks are cut and bound together. Leave them upright to dry and then thresh out the fruit. The straw is just the crushed dry stalks.

Actions—nervine tonic, anti-depressant, nutritive, demucent, vulnerary.

Indications—Oats are one of the best remedies for 'feeding' the nervous system, especialy when under stress. It is considered a specific in cases of *nervous debility* and *exhaustion* when associated with *depression.* It may be used with most of the other nervines, both relaxant and stimulatory, to strengthen the whole of the nervous system. It is also used in *general debility.* The high levels of silicic acid in the straw will explain its use as a remedy for skin conditions, especially in external applications.

Combinations—for *depression* it may be used with Scullcap and Lady's-slipper.

Caution—should not be used by people who have gluten allergies.

Dosage—1–4 g of the dried herb or oatmeal as an infusion three times a day. Porridge provides a good source.

PASQUE-FLOWER

(Anemone pulsatilla, Ranunculaceae)

Part used—aerial parts.

Collection—the stalks should be gathered at the time of flowering, which is in March or April.

Actions—sedative, analgesic, anti-spasmodic, anti-bacterial.

Indications—Pasque-flower is an excellent relaxing nervine for use in problems relating to *nervous tension* and *spasm* in the reproductive system. It may be used with safety in the relief of *painful periods (dysmenorrhoea), ovarian pain* and *painful conditions of the testes.* Pasque-flower has valuable properties in easing *pre-menstrual tension,* and anxiety associated with the *menopause.* It may be used to reduce *tension reactions* and *headaches* associated with them. It will help *insomnia* and general *overactivity.*

The anti-bacterial actions give this herb a role in treating infections that affect the skin, especially *boils*. It is similarly useful in the treatment of *respiratory infections* and *asthma*. The oil or tincture will ease *earache*.

Combinations—for *painful periods* it will combine well with Cramp-bark. For *skin conditions* it combines with Echinacea.

Caution—do not use the fresh plant!

Dosage—0.1–0.3 g of the dried leaves three times a day.

PASSION-FLOWER
(*Passiflora incarnata*, Passifloraceae)

Part used—dried leaves.

Collection—if the foliage alone is to be collected, this should happen just before the flowers bloom, between May and July. The foliage may be collected with the fruit after flowering. It should be dried in the shade.

Actions—sedative, hypnotic, anti-spasmodic, anodyne.

Indications—Passion-flower is the herb of choice for treating *intransigent insomnia*. It aids the transition into a restful sleep without any 'narcotic' hangover. It may be used wherever an anti-spasmodic is required, e.g. in *Parkinson's disease, seizures* and *hysteria*. It can be very effective in *nerve pain* such as *neuralgia* and the viral infection of nerves called *shingles*. It may be used in *asthma* where there is much spasmodic activity, especially when there is associated tension.

Combinations—for *insomnia* it will combine well with Valerian, Hops and Jamaican Dogwood.

Dosage—0.5–1 g (a teaspoonful) as an infusion drunk three times a day. For use

at night make a much stronger tea.

PEPPERMINT
(*Mentha piperita*, Labiatae)

Part used—aerial parts.

Collection—the aerial parts are collected just before the flowers open.

Actions—carminative, anti-spasmodic, aromatic, diaphoretic, anti-emetic, nervine, antiseptic, analgesic.

Indications—Peppermint is one of the best carminative agents available. It has a relaxing effect on the visceral muscles, anti-flatulent properties and stimulates bile and digestive juice secretion, all of which help to explain its value in relieving *intestinal colic, flatulent dyspepsia* and other associated conditions. The volatile oil acts as a mild anaesthetic to the stomach wall, which allays feelings of *nausea* and the desire to *vomit*. It helps to relieve the *vomiting of pregnancy* and *travel sickness*. Peppermint plays a role in the treatment of *ulcerative colitis* and *Crohn's disease*. Peppermint is most valuable in the treatment of *fevers* and especially *colds* and *influenza*. As an inhalant it can be used as a temporary treatment of *nasal catarrh*. Where *migraine headaches* are associated with the digestion, this herb may be used. As a nervine it acts as a tonic, easing *anxiety, tension, hysteria,* etc. In *painful periods (dysmenorrhea)* it relieves the pain and eases associated tension. Externally it may be used to relieve *itching* and *inflammations*.

Combinations—for *colds* and *influenza* it may be used with Boneset, Elder Flowers and Yarrow.

Dosage—1–4 g (1–2 teaspoonsful) of the dried leaves used as an infusion three times a day.

ROSEMARY

(Rosemarinus officinalis, Labiatae)

Part used—leaves and twigs.

Collection—the leaves may be gathered throughout the summer but are at their best during flowering time.

Actions—carminative, aromatic, anti-spasmodic, anti-depressive, antiseptic, rubefacient, parasiticide.

Indications—Rosemary acts as a circulatory and nervine stimulant, which in addition to the toning and calming effect on the digestion makes it a remedy that is used where psychological tension is present. This may show for instance as *flatulent dyspepsia, headache* or *depression* associated with *debility*. It may be of use in *migraine, palpitations* and other signs of nervous tension. Externally it may be used to ease *muscular pain, sciatica* and neuralgia. It acts as a stimulant to the hair follicles and may be used in *premature baldness*. The oil is most effective here.

Combinations—for *depression* it may be used with Scullcap, Kola and Oats.

Dosage—1–4 g (1–2 teaspoonsful) of the dried herb as an infused tea three times a day. It is most effective when used over a period of at least three weeks.

ST JOHN'S WORT

(Hypericum perforatum, Hypericaceae)

Part used—aerial parts.

Collection—the entire plant above ground should be collected when in flower and dried as quickly as possible.

Actions—nervine tonic, astringent, local anodyne.

Indications—taken internally, St John's Wort has a sedative and pain-reducing effect, which gives it a place in the treatment of *neuralgia, anxiety, tension* and similar problems. Where these problems have been going on long enough to produce *debility* and *fatigue*, St John's Wort will prove invaluable. It is especially regarded as a herb to use where there are menopausal changes triggering *irritability* and *anxiety*. It is recommended, however, that it be not used when there is marked depression. In addition to *neuralgic pain*, it will ease *fibrositis, sciatica* and *rheumatic pain*. Externally it is a valuable healing and anti-inflammatory remedy. As a lotion it will speed the healing of *wounds* and *bruises, varicose veins* and *mild burns*. The oil is especially useful for the healing of *sunburn, neuralgia* and *fibrositis*.

Dosage—1–4 g (1–2 teaspoonsful) used as an infusion drunk three times a day. The tincture has all the value of the dried plant. Another herb that achieves best results when used over a period of time.

SCULLCAP

(Scutellaria laterifolia, Labiatae)

Part used—aerial parts.

Collection—the whole of the aerial parts should be collected late in the flowering period during August and September.

Actions—nervine tonic, sedative, anti-spasmodic.

Indications—Scullcap is perhaps the most widely relevant nervine available to us in the materia medica. It relaxes states of *nervous tension* and *anxiety*, whilst at the same time renewing and revivifying the central nervous system. It has a specific use in the treatment of *seizure* and *hysterical states* as well as *epilepsy*. It may be used in all *exhausted, debilitated* or *depressed* conditions. It can be used with complete safety in the easing of *pre-menstrual tension.*

Combinations—it combines well with Valerian.

Dosage—1–4 g (1–2 teaspoonsful) used as an infused tea three times a day. The tincture is of similar value.

SIBERIAN GINSENG
(Eleutherococcus senticosus, Araliaceae)
Part used—root.

Actions—adaptogen, circulatory stimulant, vasodilator, similar in action to Asiatic Ginseng.

Indications—a valuable remedy for improving stamina when the person is under excessive physical and mental demands. It will improve vitality in the face of *exhaustion, debility* and *depression.* There appears to be an increase in resistance to more generalized stresses such as *infections, disease* and *ageing.* There is some evidence that the early stages of *arteriosclerosis* can be reversed.

Dosage—0.2–1 g of the root three times a day.

SQUAW-VINE
(Mitchelia repens, Rubiaceae)
Part used—aerial parts.

Actions—nervine tonic, uterine tonic.

Indications—whilst primarily finding use in facilitating *labour* and easing *delivery* in labour, Squaw-vine is an excellent remedy for *painful periods, nervous debility* and *exhaustion* and *general irritability.*

Dosage—1–4 g (1–2 teaspoonsful)

drunk as an infused tea three times a day.

SWEET FLAG
(Acorus calamus, Araceae)
Part used—rhizome.

Action—carminative, relaxant.

Indications—specific for *over-acidity of the stomach* and *peptic ulceration.* As a relaxing nervine with marked carminative properties it will ease intestinal *colic* and *flatulence.*

Dosage—0.5–3 g of the rhizome three times a day as a decoction.

VALERIAN
(Valeriana officinalis, Valerianaceae)
Part used—rhizome and roots.

Collection—the roots are unearthed in the late autumn. Clean thoroughly and dry in the shade.

Actions—sedative, hypnotic, antispasmodic, hypotensive, carminative.

Indications—Valerian is one of the most useful relaxing nervines that is available to us. This fact is recognized by orthodox medicines as is shown by its inclusion in many pharmacopoeias as a sedative. It may safely be used to reduce *tension* and *anxiety, over-excitability* and *hysterical states.* It is an effective aid in *insomnia,* producing a natural healing sleep. As an anti-spasmodic herb it will aid in the relief of *cramp* and *intestinal colic* and will also be useful for the *cramps* and *pain of periods.* As a pain reliever it is most indicated where that pain is associated with tension. Valerian can help in *migraine* and *rheumatic pain.*

Combinations—for the relief of *tension* it will combine most effectively with Scullcap. For *insomnia* it can be combined with Passion-flower and Hops. For the treatment of *cramps* it will work well with Cramp-bark.

Dosage—1–4 g (1–2 teaspoonsful) of the dried root made into an infusion and drunk three times a day. This root is used as an infusion because of its rich content of volatile oils.

VERVAIN

(*Verbena officinalis*, Labiatae)

Part used—aerial parts.

Collection—the herb should be collected just before the flowers open, usually in July. Dry quickly.

Actions—nervine tonic, sedative, antispasmodic, diaphoretic, possible galactagogue, hepatic.

Indications—Vervain is a herb that will strengthen the nervous system whilst relaxing any tension and stress. It can be used to ease *depression* and *melancholia*, especially when this follows illness such as influenza. Vervain may be used to help in *seizure* and *hysteria*. As a diaphoretic it can be used in the early stages of *fevers*. As a hepatic remedy it will be of help in *inflammation of the gall-bladder* and *jaundice*. It may be used as a mouthwash against *caries* and *gum disease*.

Combinations—in the treatment of *depression* it may be used with Scullcap, Oats and Lady's-slipper.

Dosage—1–4 g (1–2 teaspoonsful) drunk as an infused tea three times a day.

WILD LETTUCE

(*Lactuca virosa*, Compositae)

Part used—dried leaves.

Collection—the leaves should be gathered in June and July.

Actions—sedative, anodyne, hypnotic.

Indications—the latex of the Wild Lettuce was at one time sold as 'Lettuce Opium', naming the use of this herb quite well! It is a valuable remedy for use in *insomnia*, *restlessness* and *excitability* (especialy in children) and other manifestations of an overactive nervous system. As an anti-spasmodic it can be used as part of a holistic treatment of *whooping cough* and dry, irritated coughs in general. It will relieve colic pains in the gut and uterus and so may be used in *painful periods*. It will ease muscular pains related to *rheumatism*. It has been used as an aphrodisiac.

Combinations—for *irritable coughs* it may be used with Wild Cherry Bark. For *insomnia* it combines with Valerian and Pasque-flower.

Dosage—0.5–3 g (1–2 teaspoonsful) of the dried herb three times a day, or a stronger tea at night.

WORMWOOD

(*Artemisia absinthium*, Compositae)

Part used—leaves or flowering tops.

Collection—the leaves and flowering tops are gathered at the end of the flowering period between July and September.

Actions—bitter tonic, carminative, anthelmintic, anti-inflammatory.

Indications—traditionally, Wormwood has been used in a wide range of conditions, most of which have been vindicated by analysis of the herb. It is primarily used as a bitter and therefore has the effect of stimulating and invigorating the whole of the digestive process. It may be used where there is *indigestion*, especially when due to a powerful remedy in the treatment of *worm infestations*, especially *roundworm* and *pinworm*. It may also be used to help the body deal with *fever* and *infections*. Due to the general tonic action it will be of benefit in many diverse conditions because it benefits the body in general.

Dosage—1–2 g (a teaspoonful) of the dried herb drunk as an infused tea three times a day, or the equivalent in tincture form.

Select Bibliography

Herbals

British Herbal Medicine Association *British Herbal Pharmacopoeia*, Volumes 1, 2 and 3.

Christopher, John R. *School of Natural Healing* BiWorld (1976)

Grieve, M. *A Modern Herbal* Dover Publications (1931)

Hoffmann, David L. *The Holistic Herbal* Findhorn (1983)

Lust, John *The Herb Book* Bantam Books (1974)

Parvati, Jeannine *Hygieia* Wildwood House (1978)

Potter's New Cyclopaedia of Botanical Drugs Health Science Press (1975)

Priest & Priest *Herbal Medication* Fowler (1982)

General Books of Help and Advice

Cox, Tom *Stress* Macmillan Press (1983)

LeShan, Lawrence *Holistic Health* Turnstone Press (1982)

Rowe, Dorothy *Depression – A way out of your prison* Routledge & Kegan Paul (1983)

Shuttle, Penelope and Redgrove, Peter *The Wise Wound, Eve's Curse and Every Woman* Gollancz (1978)

Simonton, Carl and Stephanie *Getting Well Again* Bantam (1980)

Which? Magazine *Living with Stress* Consumer's Association (1982)

Index